THE SUITCASE

Caitlin Press Inc.
8100 Alderwood Road, Halfmoon Bay, BC V0N 1Y1
www.caitlin-press.com

Text design by Vici Johnstone
Front cover design by Michael Despotovic
Cover photo by Yeshi Kangrang, from Unsplash
Printed in Canada

Caitlin Press Inc. acknowledges financial support from the Government of Canada and the Canada Council for the Arts, and the Province of British Columbia through the British Columbia Arts Council and the Book Publisher's Tax Credit.

Library and Archives Canada Cataloguing in Publication

Livingston, Becky, 1958-, author
The suitcase and the jar : travels with a daughter's ashes
    / Becky Livingston.

ISBN 978-1-987915-74-7 (softcover)
        1. Livingston, Becky, 1958-. 2. Livingston, Becky, 1958- — Travel. 3. Parental grief. 4. Mothers and daughters. I. Title.

BF575.G7L587 2018   155.9'37   C2018-902199-3

The Suitcase
&
the Jar

travels with a daughter's ashes

Becky Livingston

CAITLIN PRESS

Praise for *The Suitcase & the Jar*

What an honour to be invited to travel alongside Becky Livingston as she deftly navigates the daunting terrain of grief and loss. Carrying our stories can feel like painfully heavy baggage. Becky's journey is literally one of lessening her load, while the uncharted territory she explores begins to heal her heart. A writing style that is rich, warm and honest left me not wanting her travels to end. *The Suitcase & the Jar* helps us understand that when we fully experience the loss of someone we love deeply, we discover a part of ourselves.

—Katy Hutchison,
author of *Walking After Midnight*

Becky Livingston's travelogue of grief is tender, searing and seeded with hard-won bits of wisdom. Joy is possible in the world of grief, she tells us. Claim it. This is a book not only about surviving profound loss, but about relearning how to embrace life fully.

—Nancy Horan,
author of *Under the Wide and Starry Sky*

From the ashes a fire shall be woken
— J.R.R. Tolkien

Contents

Often you wake, not knowing where you are.

A tingling panic. *Where the hell am I?*

Piece together your movements from the night before. Heart thumps, loud and fast. Is that the bedroom door? Bathroom door? A closet?

Sometimes it hits hardest when jet lag kicks in; memory warps across time zones. Other times, bouts of late-night drinking add to the confusion.

Isn't this to be expected when you sleep in a foreign bed or in another person's house? If there's a strange sound, terror is amplified tenfold.

798 days. Crossing borders, skipping seasons, changing hemispheres.

You exhale slowly. Palm on chest, you listen for the pounding to settle, as if to recalibrate some circadian rhythm.

Here I am. Here I am.

CHAPTER 1

THE JAR

People called me courageous for leaving like I did. It's not how I saw it. I saw it as an act of self-love and preservation. Faith in second chances.

No, the great courage, The Great Courage was unscrewing the lid.

At first it was disarming.

The trick is to not let it stop you. Fear makes your hands shake. Courage makes you do it. Practice, if you can call it that, makes it less traumatic. But the first times were the worst.

You.

Open.

Touch.

Feel.

Her.

Let her go.

Let her go.

Gone.

You.

Walk away.

I thought if I could do this, I could do anything.

Just thinking about it, the surge igniting my heart, the pounding against my ribs, my legs flooded with adrenaline.

I practised first, ran a mental movie of the scene to come. The jar. Which pocket? Left? Right? Zipped open my handbag and took a look. Yep, there it was.

How much to leave?

Sometimes, just a pinch. Other times, the entire jar was emptied all at once. The amount was proportionate with my love of a place. Sometimes no place felt like a right place. Bukit Timah, a nature reserve recommended by a traveller friend, wasn't beautiful at all. I just wanted to say, "She's been to Singapore."

Privacy was best. No one to stare at the woman crouching down, muttering to herself, as if she'd absconded some illicit substance and was now full of self-recriminations. No one around to hear the whispered commentary, "Hey babe, here we are," as if she'd like to know.

She'd like to know.

A home in Edgemont Village in North Vancouver was my very first house-sit. On the back deck was a potted rose, the fragrance peaking at dusk. I watched, over two weeks, the peach bud become a full bloom, the velvet unfolding. Each evening, reclining on the lounge chair, I'd shift my glance: rose — jar — rose. Should I? Now? Like contemplating any covert operation, like shoplifting or masturbating outdoors, it required adequate planning: a furtive glance at the neighbours' bedroom window, at gaps in the length of hedge.

It felt slightly criminal, poking my sticky fork into the dirt, smooshing her bones an inch deep. Her fertility never as she imagined.

There's no mistaking that watched feeling. The fear was that I'd be caught off-guard like that man in the bushes at Zion National Park years ago.

"Do you know what the time is?" I'd asked. He'd stared at me through gold aviator sunglasses, frantic, his face growing flush pink until from where I sat, sprawled out on that rock above him, I noticed his hand full of himself, pumping rhythmically until I looked away. Finally.

Cities were a challenge. No privacy. I'd hoped to leave some at London's Borough Market (like many twenty-three-year-olds, she loved markets). Or throw some off London Bridge into the Thames. On Hampstead Heath, the epic view of London's skyline, there were still too many people.

Wind caused all kinds of problems. In the summer of 2010, five months after she died, I'd taken her to Dun Aengus on the Aran Island of Inishmore. An ancient stone fort built on the edge of a hundred-metre cliff.

I was there, with thirty others, on a poetry retreat with David Whyte. Many of us chose to lie out on the edge. Make vows for a future life. The first step was to cast away something into the hungry waves below. I knew what mine would be.

Pressed against icy Druidic rock, we'd lain prone. Arms outstretched. Pummelled by the violent Atlantic winds. I could feel the jar pressing into the bone of my right hip.

Saturated with bravado and sea spray, I'd looked over the sheer drop beyond my wet, whitening fingers when a fresh cracking wind billowed open my hood, snatching my breath. I knew then she'd stay in my pocket. Ashes are ashes. There's no telling where they might end up.

Quiet. I liked it quiet too. When sounds were muted there was just her burned bones rattling gently against the clear sides of the plastic jar, beneath the green lid. Sometimes I held it up to the light. How much was left?

When I found "the spot," I'd stare with tunnel vision. The whole world disappeared. I'd go deaf. So this was the sound that five litres of blood must make, pumping into the heart all at once. The wing-beat swells of grief like glugging wine from a bottle. The ringing in my ears, stepping forward, weaker now, as I contemplated what I was about to do.

In the silence that followed, I listened differently. Time stopped.

When it was all done I'd look at the grey dust, sometimes with a pleasurable rush: those silvery flecks. What *is* that? Other times, disgust. A young woman shaped to nothingness. One I made. Held on to. Then had to let go.

Would she make it through a winter undisturbed or be discovered by a child who might poke her with a stick? That's why I hid her. And why, perhaps, the stillness of land was my least favourite place. Dirt brought her ashes into relief. What was left visible, I erased with my fingertips. Remote spots. Speedy exits. They were the best. Take note.

No one could find, or define, her there.

Decorum was a factor. How long should I stay after it was done? Too quick felt irreverent. It meant having to talk to her in my head as I turned and walked away. That was never quite right.

"C'mon, Mum, can't you stay a moment, tell me where I am? I'm counting on you."

Yet one time, I could hardly wait to let her go.

It was early December 2011 when I'd arrived in Perth, an oppressive thirty-seven degrees Celsius when I gathered up my towel, sunscreen and the jar, and walked down to the beach at Ocean Reef.

The ocean blazed blue. An endless expanse of cream white sand. Nothing but sand and sea for miles. But I'm getting ahead of myself. By the time I reached the beach she was all gone.

The pathway from the road. It led me in. I heard it, the beckoning ocean, and I was already unscrewing the lid and pouring her into my right hand, laughing as she spilled between my fingers. Onto my flip-flops.

No, I didn't care if anyone heard me yahooing.

Australia, I love you! It's so good to be back.

I didn't care if anyone saw me leave a little there, at the base of a fence post, a little here, under the wire. I didn't care if anyone saw me turn around, stumbling back along the path, turn around, go back again, and repeat the entire operation. I was a drunken farmer sowing seeds in the sand. Drunk on bliss. I wanted her to know above everything else that my journey was the result of her love.

CHAPTER 2

CRUISING AT ALTITUDE

Unless you looked closely, you wouldn't have noticed the scar. Her natural waves camouflaged it well. Shaped like the letter C, it scored a line that severed her scalp, tucked neatly behind her left ear where the skin was still a little pink. Inflamed.

There were no tears at the airport, only nervous laughter and mild restraint. Hugs were big and firm; kisses quick. *Safe travels. Love you. Have fun.* Five months in New Zealand. Alone.

"Phone me once a week."

February 2005, with the all-clear from the doctors, she was off. Some questioned our decision, her condition so raw. My partner, Bob, his arm around my waist, pulled me in tight to his side, kissed my head.

"She'll be fine."

She waved her passport high above her head. Thrust out from the top, her boarding pass.

There she goes. My eighteen-year-old daughter, Rachel. Bristling with promise. A young woman who'd mastered the art of living with uncertainty. With questions that have no answers. The big one: How long would radiation keep the brain tumour from returning? A year? Two years? Ten?

For Rachel, it would be five.

Let me tell you something about her.

She was happiest travelling.

And something else:

She belongs to the world now, not to me.

I like to think she's playing in the shifting sands, caught between your children's toes or carried home in a castle-shaped pail. All of us carrying her away.

I like to think she's cruising now at altitude. Snatched away in the wind. Taken by the ocean. Spanning the globe. My intrepid traveller, shape-shifting. Miraculous in flight. Her dancing feet discovering unexplored countries. Dust motes in the moonlight. Chasing light. At airports, where everyone's moving on. And yes, even beneath a spiral stairwell high up in the Himalayas. That's where I need her to be. Unconfined. Released to so many unknowns who'll know her in ways I won't. Places I carried her ashes, places I may well have ignored without them.

The image of her face. She's lying in bed. Her final weeks. Conviction in her voice.

"Ramp!"

"Ramp?"

"Yes."

"You want a ramp to get you out the house?"

"Yes!"

I couldn't tell her that these things take time. But her intention was clear. She needed to feel the air on her face again, feel her body moving. The dream, all along, to be free.

So I travelled for her, and with her. Rachel reduced to almost nothing, and me, to the contents of a suitcase. I had no idea how hard it would be, how much terrain I would have to explore to understand the world without my daughter. The world as it was now.

Eighteen months after she died — it was time.

CHAPTER 3

THE LONE MARKER

How do you pack a suitcase to hold the contents of your life?

Stand in your bedroom.

Look around.

Which items are essential for a year away?

Will fit into one suitcase without exceeding the weight limit?

Then open up your bathroom cabinets and do the same.

Your desk too, if you have one.

Then your bookcase.

What, without question, needs to come with you?

Do you take a book? Two? More? A journal?

How many pairs of shoes? If you're not sure where you're going, do you take sandals *and* hiking boots?

Jewelry?

A talisman to keep you safe?

Knowing what brings you comfort, is key.

Pico Iyer says, "Home lies in the things you carry with you everywhere and not the ones that tie you down."

Rachel gave up everything. Now it was my turn.

Her final words, "follow your heart," impossible to ignore. From that time onward, I was to discover how.

Giving up my apartment was easy. Quitting my job was easier. Taking control of *something* propelled me through those final weeks at work. I could restart my life, just as soon as I got on that plane.

Other than a confirmed two-month stay in a tiny Spanish village, there was no agenda. After that I let the winds carry me away in a kind of blind surrender. To have a plan would have been a mistake. I had to feel my way through this.

"Isn't it foolish for a fifty-three-year-old woman to just abandon her job and head off overseas without a plan? My guess is you won't find what you're looking for in some far-off land," said a friend. "What you're looking for is already in you. Your life is already as it should be."

A fan of Eckhart Tolle? In my gut I sensed that far-off lands would offer me the space to see beyond what I looked past at home. I was reminded of the line from Eric Weiner's *The Geography of Bliss*: "Where we are is vital to who we are."

Lose yourself to find yourself. It's what ancient wisdom advocates. I was exhausted by "my story." Living incognito was exactly what I needed.

The journey I envisioned was more than just fulfilling my daughter's dying wish to keep travelling; it was the need to see the world through her eyes and to know her courage and her joy. Only on a vast canvas could I come to this knowing. To get to where she was, without encumbrances.

I decide that my daughters will go with me everywhere: the ashes of one — *not all of them,* just enough to fill a medium-sized Ziploc bag — and a photograph of the other.

It's amazing how much I need to leave behind.

I hide the Ziploc inside an old Maggie B makeup bag with a zipper closure and a popper-down flap. The quilted lining is all ripped up and it crinkles. Then there's the jar. Barely two inches tall and an inch wide, the plastic jar is the pocket-sized home for my daughter's ashes. Deserving Thyme bath salts, washed down a drain at a hotel on Vancouver Island, were replaced with her ashes; it slips easily into my Baggalini handbag. Beside my camera. My passport.

Ashes take up little space: heavy, but easily transportable. In the pieces of her burned body, there is a paradox that comforts me.

You can only take her if you're willing to let her go.

When the children were back at school and the airfares more affordable, I flew away.

It's late September 2011 when I land at Mallorca's Palma airport. 6 p.m. Well past the scheduled arrival time.

The landlady had typed out detailed driving instructions to her house, single-spaced: "Take an early flight. It's better than arriving in the semi-dark or at nighttime. Just a thought!"

Here's what I knew: Her home in Llucalcari had no hot water, no washer (or dryer) and the bathroom was outside. A nude beach was a twenty-minute walk from the village. The neighbours were friendly but spoke only Spanish; and a brilliant writer and linguist, Nicole, lived across the street.

No great fan of solitude, I knew that to completely remove myself from people would be a mistake. Being part of something was preferable to nothing. But could I ever be still enough to find out? Is this why I chose Mallorca's smallest village?

There it is, on the baggage carousel: the Suitcase, with Rachel's navy and white bandana knotted to the red handle. A small, but essential, token of her presence. Proof, she's travelling.

She'd owned the bandana for years but wore it only after that first surgery in 2002, when her long dark hair resembled a bird's nest: dry, bloody tangles, wiry and wild and voluminous, as if someone in the operating room had spent hours back-combing it. Three days post-surgery I'd braided her hair into eight or nine mini-braids. It took the better part of an afternoon. They stuck out of her head like old rope gnawed on by rodents. Her friends dropped by.

"Can we take Rachel down to London Drugs? It's only a short walk."

"Sure," I said. "You up for that, Rach?"

Already Rachel had folded the bandana neatly in half and was holding it above her head. I watched it touch down on her scalp, gently like a tablecloth floating to land, the air blown away. She tied the two ends at the base of her neck, once then twice, adjusting it to hide the pink flesh and the one staple just above her left ear.

"How's that?" she asked. "Can you see any staples?"

"Perfect," I said. She looked amazing.

"Thanks, Mum, see you later."

How quickly the young heal, I thought. How fortunate to have a daughter so self-assured and nonplussed by all that's happened. I loved this about her.

Llucalcari, Mallorca, a one-street village nestled along the north coast, warrants a name on a Google map but not on a road sign in the real world. The sun is setting as I pull out of the Repsol gas station with a full tank. I kick off my flip-flops and drive toward the silhouette of black mountains.

Valldemossa, the first village en route to my new home, is lit like a dream hamlet for Christmas. I roll down my window, the night air still so warm.

Shortly thereafter, things change: the breeze is cooler, the blackness to my left must be the ocean at night. I can smell it, feel it: the sound of waves melding to one gigantic undulating sea. I want to stop, but there's no place to pull over.

Around a deep curve come the lights of Deia. Swags of twinkling lights above the back deck of a restaurant. I drive through the village; easy bodies in floating fabrics and skimpy sandals press gently against the stone walls to let my car pass. The pavement is only wide enough for one.

Llucalcari, I know, must be close. Very close.

On I go, navigating hairpin bends in the pitch of night, talking to myself. Fifteen minutes later it's clear I've missed my turn. That's not so bad; the trick is to find a place to turn around. I begin to laugh. It's exactly what Rachel would've done, were she sitting beside me. Then I start to cry.

I have to drive miles out of my way before I can turn and get back on track.

A bus stop is the lone identifying marker for Llucalcari. The descent into the village is perilous.

Down — brake. Down — brake. Down.

This is followed by a "No Entry" lane, the only way in or out. With exacting precision, I maneuver the Fiat into a teensy parking space, one of just three in the village, and congratulate myself.

With careful instructions arrogantly ignored on the back seat, I climb out of the rental car and begin searching for my *caserio*.

Houses are glued together like a fortress wall. Yellow bulbs high, high up illuminate the cul-de-sac with faint shadows. There's a church. It's locked and barred. My house, No. 13, is attached to the church. Built in 1688, The Virgin of the Helpless.

I wiggle the key into the massive door. It opens with a clunk and a creak. The musty smell is overwhelming, tells the story of its years. I stand frozen in the pitch black. Shiver.

I reach out with my flashlight, find the kitchen in the far back. Dishes are still draining beside the sink, a long granite slab. Two terracotta bowls (one, I assume, for washing, the other for rinsing) are upturned beneath the cold tap, which juts out from the wall.

"There's a kettle if you need hot water," she'd written in a recent email.

A row of cold beer is lined up in the fridge door. I pull back the tab from one and head back outside. The village is asleep.

The sea is only a suggestion in the distance. Against the silence, I hear it gently lapping.

The house has three floors. On the top floor is the art studio. It's where I spend most of my days, because it's the only room that gets any air or light. And light, I know, is an antidote to depression. Opening all three windows I feel *something* moving.

The north window looks out onto a sea of glazed turquoise, and the sky, like those in Rachel's photos from Greece, is a Santorini blue. Across the room, a smaller window looks out over the terracotta tiles of the church roof, the afternoon light catching the curves. Beyond, but not far away, is the craggy backbone of Mallorca: the Serra de Tramuntana mountain range. Most people I know would give anything to call this place home for two months. I try to like it. But there is no respite inside of me.

The bathroom outside, at night I pee in a bucket in my bedroom.

Nicole lives across the street from my *caserio*. A native Mallorcan born to a French mother and an El Salvadorian father, she's both multilingual and beautiful; a prolific reader, writer and smoker. Her novel, *Cartas / Selected Letters*, a translation of Emily Dickinson's poems and letters, made Spain's Top 10 bestseller list.

Local children come and go from her casa, hoping to improve their English under her tutelage. I'm certain she tutors solely to pay the bills. Her live-in boyfriend has difficulty holding down a job.

She was topless when we first met. Perched on a giant boulder, her knees drawn in to her bare chest, she was reading a book. I noticed her vertebrae bulging down the length of her tanned back all the way to her red bikini bottoms. She was smoking a cigarette, using the same hand to brush aside the fine dark hair from her face. There was no fat on her girlish frame nor, I realized, on any locals with the agility to scale the perilous slope down to the water's edge. Everyone was topless. It's how many people "take the sun" on this side of the Atlantic. I found it difficult not to stare.

I ask Nicole to be my Spanish tutor. She accepts. Twice a week we sit outside at her table beneath the grapevine trellis, stray cats at our feet, and speak only Spanish.

By the second class I discover *un tumor cerebral* took the life of her sixteen-year-old cousin.

"Do you want to meet again next week?" she asks, rubbing her hands together and blowing on them for warmth. "It's getting cool out here, isn't it?"

"Is it?"

By the third week I'm certain she's bored with our sessions. I'm always on time; she's not. I can tell she's just stubbed out a cigarette. Her fingers are cold and twitchy and they smell. Am I that bad at Spanish, I wonder?

The next class is our last.

"I need to leave Llucalcari." Nicole speaks to me in English. "Sergio, my boyfriend, has been making physical threats. So I shall move to Palma. I need you, as a friend."

Nicole's aloofness I realized was not about me. And it struck me just then, perhaps only then, that grief isn't exclusive to dying.

She'd tied up her books into piles of fifty, each a metre high. I marvelled at the precision of her perfectly knotted twine.

"May I store some in your house? My car's completely full."

"No worries," I said.

We carried them, nine piles, across the street to my house and up to the office on the second floor. The fine string left imprints on my fingers.

"I'll come to pick them up another day."

For centuries, life by the sea has been best where doors open onto back decks or up to rooftops. Not the medieval dark of a home wedged between a derelict church and Spanish neighbours whose TV screen is always moving.

My house was everything I was: dark, hollow, solitary and heavy. No deck or balcony. Just a small secluded space out back with two stone sinks built into the wall. This is where I carry my clothes to wash them. My palms blistered with all the wringing, the rawness of opposing turns.

Three clotheslines zigzag overhead. Only at the height of day does the sunlight touch my wet clothes. Sometimes I sit on a chair beneath the clotheslines and peel the skin from an orange, letting the juice dribble on the stone.

Across the street are four homes attached to each other. Each has a back door that opens out onto a communal deck of patchwork slate. Above, a string of twinkling lights loops around a trellis. Beat-up wicker chairs pulled in together make for easy conversation. There's Fanny and Phil from Belgium; Nicole, my Spanish tutor; and occasionally Olc, the Barcelonian entrepreneur who owns all four properties. And there's me, for a while. But I don't live here, and I feel like an imposter. I live in the house across the street.

"See ya later." I wave goodbye, heave open my front door and climb the cold stone stairs, two flights, my breathing laboured, up to the top floor, and lean out the front window. I hear them laughing over there.

Why didn't you stay? This is Europe, not Canada. But I don't, and I don't know why. Only that hovering between grief and engagement is an unsteady dance. In this home it requires little effort to stay lonely. And it's lonely to live in the world and be afraid. Bone deep.

I roll out the yoga mat alongside the crack where last week I'd watched a scorpion scuttle away. Both of us froze, unsure of who should be more afraid. *Vicky Cristina Barcelona* is my yoga soundtrack. I play the songs in order so I know what track comes next. It's all I ever play these days.

No one phones me. It's fine. I like it that way. A ringing phone can mean catastrophe. My daughter Charlotte doesn't call. Nor do my friends from Canada. The call I'm dreading is the one from my sister Debbie in England, telling me that one of our parents is ill and requires care. Afraid that, unemployed, I'll be the natural choice to step in, having proven myself a caregiver to the dying. I don't know what I would do.

February 13, 2006, ten days after Bob and I moved into our new home, he'd called.

"Hey," he croaked.

"Where are you?"

"I'm in the hospital."

"Hospital? I don't understand."

"I've had a seizure."

"What do you mean?"

"There's something in my head. I've got something in my head."

"What?"

"Something in my head, like Rachel."

"What!"

"I didn't want to call you at school." His voice parched. "I didn't want you to find out that way. Not again."

Rachel was still sitting at the kitchen table, enjoying a bowl of Mr. Noodles.

"What's happened?" she said.

"Bob. He's in hospital. He's had a seizure."

I threw jeans on over my yoga pants, snatched up my fleece and slammed the door shut. I thought the glass might break. I'd forgotten how easily it rattled. How I'd need to be gentle with the old thing until we replaced it.

Rachel was already in the car.

What did he mean? *Something in his head.* Another brain tumour would be too cruel.

A faded green robe was stretched taut across his broad chest, too tiny for the heft of his six-foot-two frame. His tongue, swollen three times its normal size. I saw the bite marks, a dotted line scoring his tongue into two parts. "A self-inflicted bite is common during seizures," said the nurse.

The neurologist said, "I think it'd be better if your daughter left the room."

"Trust me. She can handle it."

"I'll wait outside," said Rachel. "It's okay."

The doctor scraped the metal curtain rings across the metal bar. I watched the folds of pale plastic wafting in the breeze of moving bodies. An illusion of privacy, inside what?

Everyone heard him say, "It's a brain tumour."

A daughter diagnosed with a brain tumour was, I thought, the worst thing that could happen. Much like a fortunate player in *Survivor* who'd endured some great challenge, I thought I had immunity.

In the spring of 2004, two years after Rachel was diagnosed with a brain tumour, I met Bob. By year end he'd moved in.

"How wonderful," said my friends. "You deserve a break. Someone to love you, help you through everything with Rachel." I'd bristle. Doesn't everyone deserve to be happy?

After living together for a year, we got engaged, we bought a house: the perfect fixer-upper for Bob, a carpenter, to renovate. Ten days after we moved in — Bob, Rachel and I — he was diagnosed with an aggressive brain cancer: a glioblastoma multiforme (GBM). Six months later he was dead.

"It's not fair," said friends. "You don't deserve this."

Most of us consider it "fair" that we experience some good and bad in a lifetime, but not too much of either. Winning the lottery twice, or two brain tumours in one family. You can't rationalize it. You can't make sense of why certain things happen to certain people. You question your vulnerability, your fate or ill-fate. You think you know the shape of your life but one day the whole fucking thing falls apart. The sensation was that I'd tripped some wire; been singled out.

None of us are immune. The notion that life is fair is an illusion asserted by parents, teachers and politicians to keep us compliant. Except I thought I was. Instead, I got a huge broken promise.

People warn the recently bereaved. "Don't do anything foolish. Something you might regret."

Four months after Rachel died, I sold the house. An easy decision. In less than four years, a household of three had been reduced to one.

I signed a one-year lease on an upscale one-bedroom apartment in Horseshoe Bay, a fresh space, far from the familiar. It made me look like I was doing okay. I wasn't. The deepest sadness was waiting for me.

August, then September. I hid from everything. Training, I realized, for living in the shadows.

Trying to remember you
is like carrying water
in my hands a long distance
across sand.

From "Grief" by Stephen Dobyns

I got busy. It's a hand-me-down from my mother's post-war generation of "Keep Calm and Carry On," a conviction that hard work precludes one from pain.

Nothing worked. Least of all, my return to full-time teaching. What I failed to calculate, as did Roger Rosenblatt after the death of his daughter, "is the pain that increases even as one gets on with it."

It started out badly. In the recognition ceremony at my school district to honour teachers with twenty years' service, my photo and name were mismatched.

Waking up was the hardest part. Most days I struggled in to school. Because here's the thing: you can't check grief at the classroom door. Negotiating petty arguments between eight-year-olds about who stole whose pencil is dangerous territory.

Driving home, the steering wheel clenched in my vice-like grip, I'd speed along Highway No. 1, banging the heel of my hand against the perforated padding. Not a scream but a roar from deep in my belly. Even with the windows closed I was afraid of being heard. Rainy days were the worst, the wipers wagging their long black fingers against the glass. *Can't you get your shit together?*

The paradox: how to go on, without letting go? It felt like I was holding her hand but was drowning too. To save my life, I had to release the grip. Mothers don't let go.

I craved just five more minutes of sitting across from her and *then* death could have her back. My heart hurt so much sometimes I rubbed it, wondering if I might be having a heart attack.

On good days, you say to yourself, *I'm still breathing.* The bad days too.

Something had to change.

I went hiking in the woods. Sabotaging good judgment, I chose a route I'd never hiked before. Eagle Bluffs.

The sky was white on that February morning, but no path was clear. No tracks visible in the snow. In dark shadows, slippery with moss and patchy ice, I scrambled up a rock face, following the light. Two hours, I saw no one. Heard no one.

In February the light fades quickly, a hazard that catches many hikers off guard. On Vancouver's North Shore Mountains it happens all the time. I imagine a Search and Rescue team out searching for me. Me? Now there'd be a story. My despair fully exposed.

Higher and higher I climbed, as if some kind of answer was waiting at the top. Closer to the sky. A clearing?

Nobody would miss me. Not until my absence at school tomorrow morning. I relished the thought. Last week a teacher's comment had flung me into a rage. She'd touched me on the shoulder. "She's always with you," her voice, so pious. Of all the things people said, this felt the worst.

Then it happened. Lost in thought one moment, the next, I was hovering over a dizzying height. My hiking boot inches from going over.

I leaned toward the edge, looked down. My heart thumping.

Just one more step.

The drop-off was well beyond what a body could withstand were I to fall.

All this time looking down, I'd lost focus.

Rachel was gone. Bob was gone. I was alone. Completely and utterly alone. Where was "home" without them?

So this is how despair feels. A death wish and a life wish both desperate for victory.

But there's Charlotte. My living daughter. There's me.

Ankles locked. Swaying. Left. Right. There it was! A landmark. Howe Sound stretched out far below me. I could just make it out between the gaps in the trees, a spectacular but terrifying sight. I was facing north, heading in the completely wrong direction.

Down there, somewhere, was my luxurious oversized sofa, where, in the deep down-filled cushions, I'd realized the great tragedy, that "accepting" my loss meant reconciling myself to the truth: *I'd have to live life without her.* How could I give myself this permission? I didn't want to stop grieving. Grieving kept them close. Kept her close. To get on with life felt like abandoning her.

I could feel the tears rising up in me. Hot. Stinging. The wind dried them to my cheek, a tight white.

A giant branch snagged my leg, piercing the flesh of my calf through my thick hiking pants. No one heard me cry. I slid my hand inside my pants, shocked by my body's response to fear — a warm wetness between my legs.

Which way to go? Deep into the forest, or west toward the ocean far off in the distance?

Then this. Something I'd never done before or thought I ever would. I hugged a tree. A gigantic Douglas fir.

I'd read about people further up the coast who did this kind of thing to save the forests. Tree-huggers. A photograph of a woman with her palms pressed against the trunk of a giant cedar, her head lowered between her outstretched arms, had consumed one entire page of a magazine. I wasn't one of these earthy women. I didn't want to be. But some lines from a poem, suddenly remembered now:

> *Stand still. The forest knows*
> *Where you are. You must let it find you.*

From "Lost" by David Wagoner

My hot cheek against the scruffy bark, I brushed my finger-tips along the coarse, slimy grooves. It was oddly silent, as if the world heard me holding on, and was waiting.

What happened next I recall only in fragments and images. I found the helipad, took refuge in an open sky. Helipads, I realized only then, are placed in the highest locations. All have a path leading away. I followed the path.

As a mother I knew what I must do to revive my skewered heart. Keep going. Risk life for just one more day.

If Rachel's death led me to that cliff edge moment, that moment made me find my way without her.

CHAPTER 4

How Like Snowflakes

The Snowman by Raymond Briggs is a beautifully illustrated book about the life and death of a snowman. It's the kind of book that instills a love of quality children's literature in our little ones.

One Christmas, my daughters received a copy. Yet I rarely selected it as a bedtime story, hoping that by denying my own feelings about death, theirs could be avoided. A topic we could postpone forever. It forced me to reflect on my own fears about death. How, like snowflakes, we take our unique shape, we float through the world, adored, and then we're gone. I often wondered how the two children in the story who lovingly build and decorate the snowman feel as they watch its gradual demise, knowing its death is certain.

At what point does one thing become another? The snowman, a lump of frozen water? Where did Rachel end and her brain tumour begin?

It's hard to tell when the changes in her started. It's clear to me that her tumour must have been growing for some time. How old she might have been when it took up residence in her brain, who knows?

Seldom did I pick her up from Kindergarten. I waited in my car. The bell rang. The classroom door opened and children burst out, spilling down the flight of stairs and onto the playground. Rachel was often the last, or one of the last.

And I remember she looked a little shell-shocked, as if the teacher had called her back at the last moment to take home something that the other kids had already zipped inside their backpacks. It worried me. As a teacher, I knew that by five years old, a child's destiny was largely determined. And I'm ashamed to admit that I wanted her to be more on top of things.

The family vacation in Wales, at the beach at Aberystwyth, we'd headed off for ice cream: my sister and I and our six children (all under ten) in tow.

Speediness is revered in my family, in many British families. One is not to fuss over trivialities. Ice cream flavours, for example. So the deed, once begun, is executed in haste, and everyone is standing by the ice cream van, madly licking their icy treat, waiting for Rachel (aged seven) to make her selection so the money can be exchanged and we can return to our picnic spot.

"C'mon Rachel," I said. "Just pick something. Anything!" I could sense my sister Debbie's impatience because she started in on her too.

"Hurry up, Rachel," she said. "Make a decision. There's people behind us, waiting."

Was the brain tumour already growing, or was she just like any other slightly indecisive child?

Working backwards, analyzing oddities, it's what you do. Her response to the news of Princess Diana's car crash: "Cool!" (She loved Princess Diana); the year we lived in Australia, when she complained of "fuzzy feelings" in her head. "A sudden growth spurt, most likely," said the doctor, and we went with that.

In 2001 she'd see her mother and father divorce; she'd change schools, change homes.

Four months later, there's her brain tumour on a CT scan.

The secretary at Rachel's school had called the secretary at mine. It was April 9, 2002.

The school secretary appeared in the staff room, her panicked eyes searching me out.

"Sounds like an emergency," she said, transferring the call to the medical room.

"Mrs. Livingston?"

"Yes."

"Your daughter's had a grand mal seizure."

"Which one?"

"Rachel."

"She's been taken by ambulance to Lions Gate Hospital."

After the hospital mayhem, I drove over to the high school. Charlotte was waiting in the school office, "Is Dad at the hospital?"

I nodded.

"Then I'm not going." Her stony face was unrelenting.

I crouched down beside her.

"Charlotte, this isn't about you," I said gently. "It's about your sister. You have to come."

Daryl and I had separated in 1999. Not so much acrimonious, but rather lackluster. As a single father, he'd chosen to take the proverbial back seat.

"I can't afford to feed you girls dinner," he said, "let alone breakfast."

Charlotte was twelve.

"Why would Dad have told me that?" she said, fists clenched at her side.

It changed everything. Charlotte pulled away. She hid in the basement when Daryl came to the door. One day she simply ignored his knocking.

Rachel's seizure forced a change. Daryl and Charlotte, estranged for the past year, stood on opposite sides of the hospital bed, Charlotte avoiding eye contact. All eyes were on Rachel.

Rachel, I remember, looked so healthy, even vibrant, which I found odd. Her cheeks were a polished, rosy red, her eyes shone.

Daryl tried to make light of the seizure, cracking odd jokes. *Shut up. Stop the inane chatter.* Couldn't he see Charlotte squirming? Didn't he notice that she refused to look at him? How Rachel felt, I couldn't tell. "Okay" and "Fine" offered little.

We were the adults. It wasn't our time to talk. It was theirs. Rachel retold her memory of the seizure outside the school cafeteria, again and again to us and to the medical staff on duty. Charlotte shared her version: how her friends had rushed to find her, how she'd found her sister lying on the ground, and walked alongside the gurney, out to the ambulance.

Later that evening Rachel was discharged. I drove the girls home. Daryl came too. Rachel called her friends. Charlotte headed upstairs to call hers.

With so much change, Charlotte rebelled. Rachel didn't. Or didn't appear to.

At fourteen she'd joined the local church youth group. An early start to the day was not one of Rachel's strengths, but there she was heading off to church on Sunday mornings. She and her best friend, Natalie, had a crush on a guy who loved Jesus.

But after a year of praising the Lord, it wasn't a boyfriend that she saw as her gift from the Almighty. It was a brain tumour.

"Fuck God," written on the screwed-up paper in her garbage can, weeks later — that was about it.

For years Rachel lived in neutral. I was never quite sure who was there behind that smile. Her mask of calm composure, always content to observe our family's goings-on. We were the performers. And she, the appreciative audience, laughing in all the right places.

But there's no question about it. We make ourselves powerless when we pretend not to know. Anger, turned inward, does terrible things to the body.

I always wondered. Were violent inner needs breaking through? As if the brain tumour were the manifestation of her being.

Dysembryoplastic Neuroepithelial Tumour. I wrote it on the board for my students. They liked decoding long words. Some sounded it out; others practised silently, moving their lips until they felt sure.

"How do you pronounce it?"

"Dis-embryo-plastic-neuro-epith-elial tumour or DNET for short." I had it committed to memory.

"It's a benign tumour. Benign means it's slow growing. Nothing to worry about."

"How did she get it?" one student asked.

"While she was growing inside me, as an embryo. Hence the name."

It demonstrates essentially no growth over time, although very gradual increase in size has been described. Prognosis is excellent. Lesions are often incompletely resected, but tumour progression is uncommon. Complete tumour removal is associated with a very high cure rate.

It was September 2002. I liked to think my teaching friends saw me as "holding it all together." But I was wrong.

"I'm concerned about how much weight you've lost. Others are too."

Burned out, my doctor called it. She prescribed antidepressants. I took them. Then I went to see a counsellor. Told her everything. For years I needed her. She said things like, "Grief doesn't heal us, it just changes us." So I kept going back.

"Rachel's tumour lies directly below her speech cortex," explained the neurosurgeon. "It's a high-risk location. We weren't able to remove much. Less than 5 percent, just to be safe. Speech impediments aren't well accepted in the world."

He'd know. His was quite pronounced.

Six months later we sit around a dark, polished table at BC Children's Hospital, five people in white coats, Rachel and I.

"The MRI shows the tumour's grown. This shouldn't have happened were it a DNET. We think this might possibly be an oligodendroglioma, a malignant tumour. We're recommending a course of radiation."

I recall that first note in my school mailbox, a "Please Call" note ripped from the school secretary's pink pad.

"BC Cancer Agency. How can I help you?"

I hung up.

My daughter doesn't have cancer. And please don't say that word. Conjecture, surely. This, the worst of many terrible moments.

We all have moments of revelation. When something essential changes the course of our lives. It's only later that we realize it was, at the time, something we were meant to intuit.

"I'd like to propose that Rachel have another surgery," said Dr. Goddard, the radiation oncologist. "Different neurosurgeon. Different hospital. Let's hold off on the radiation."

It was the way she just stood in the doorway, our faces mere inches apart. She stared at me about five seconds too long.

"I'm so sorry."

The sadness right there in her eyes. A puppy dog sadness.

"She's such a lovely girl."

We looked across the room at Rachel. Her hair was loose with two strips pulled back like a wishbone, tied in behind. She was sixteen, luminous.

"Isn't she?" I said.

Rituals, by nature, help restore order. I'd been a runner for years. So I knew, with a marriage fallen lame many years earlier, what it took to keep the peace at home. After Rachel's diagnosis came another ritual. Lighthouse Park in West Vancouver was, for almost eight years, my go-to place. Eight years. Two surgeries. And a prognosis that changed four times.

There's a place there, in Lighthouse Park, I call my own. I doubt you'd ever find it. (Visitors tend to the well-trodden paths.) But then again I wouldn't want you to. I claimed it years ago. So I'll tell you just this much. Deep in the woods along a promontory of sloped granite is a pocket of rock, an alcove in the grey stone. My body fits inside perfectly. Everything else is water.

The second surgery is a great success.

"Dr. Toyota removed between 60 and 80 percent" said the anesthesiologist.

We were, as you can imagine, ecstatic. *It still wasn't enough. It would never be enough.* Residual brain tumour is never good.

It's February, then March, 2003. For five weeks we wait for results. Five weeks pretending to live like normal people not waiting for life-changing news. Five weeks delving into brain tumour statistics. They're grim. Average life expectancy for benign tumours: ten years. Hers, I'm certain must be different. But late at night when the house is quiet, a slither of truth creeps in. *It's very likely my daughter will die early.* She may not see her forties. Even her thirties. I can go no lower. It lasts a second or two before I click the "X" in the top left corner of the screen. Shut it down.

For years I lived with the uncertainty inflicted by the world of medicine, in the anticipation of loss. To imagine the death of your child is utterly depleting: chronic hyper-alertness, suppressed panic. You want to know how much time your child has left, so you can know how to live. Three months? Three years? There's no relief from the agony of waiting. No remedy in statistics. The range of reasonable possibilities so wide they could never tell us.

The fear peaked in the days before and after her quarterly MRIs.

"Rachel must be terrified."

"Give people and things their own life," my counsellor said.

Joan Didion said this: "The fear is for what is still to be lost."

"Good news," said Dr. Toyota. "It's a pilocytic astrocytoma. A benign tumour. Four of the five pathologists agree."

And again medicine proves itself an imperfect art. I'd not expected good news. I'd prepared myself for the other.

"It's a tumour usually found in young people. Typically, they stay in the area where they start, and don't spread. They're considered the 'most benign' of all the astrocytomas." He handed me the report:

The third specimen is received in a plastic bag labelled with patient's name and "Brain Tumour" and consists of multiple fragments of light-tan tissue with red areas measuring approximately in aggregate 1.2 x 1.2 x 0.2 cm. Date collected: Feb. 17, 2003.

The colour. The size. Her name on the bag. Where the hell did this thing come from? And how long had it been in there? Growing red and light tan?

I was never quite sure what the surgeries did to her mental functioning.

"Rachel doesn't process language like she once did," said her Grade 12 English teacher. "In Grade 10 she was a top student. These days she looks overwhelmed and rarely contributes." At home, I never noticed the change. But then you don't as a rule, when you don't want to see. "She isn't quick enough," said the manager of JJ Bean. Packing groceries at Whole Foods — a similar story.

Five years later, in December of 2008, Rachel's tumour changes. How do I know? Because she starts to say "Yes" when she means "No," or says the wrong word entirely. I try not to notice. So does she. At first we laugh about it. Then we can't.

"I try not to talk to people at work," she says. "I get my words mixed up. They'll think I'm stupid."

I notice, for the first time, the lanyard hanging around her neck, white against her black button-up shirt. The sudden focus you get before a life shifts.

She'd showed me the ID tag when she arrived home after her first day at the Pacific Press. I'd glanced quickly, on to something else.

Lanyard: a rope or cord worn around the neck, used where there is a risk of losing the object.

For almost seven years I've been afraid. Afraid this birthday, or that Christmas, or next Easter, might be the last. Rushing around in my professional life, ignoring the chaos in my inner life, where the primal fear of losing control lies. Of losing my daughter.

The fourth (and final) diagnosis of Rachel's tumour: an infiltrating glioma.

Inoperable.

Snow falls.

It sticks.

She makes snow angels.

Out there in the back garden in her new snow pants. Testing them out.

I watch her face from the deck, her eyes wide.

She's laughing, opening her mouth to catch the flakes.

I start to laugh too.

CHAPTER 5

WHO DID I TELL?

Like many Irish summer days, the sky is a blanket of grey. The Burren, in County Clare, is a place of remembering. A place that invites contemplation, yet demands absolute focus; one missed step and you're down, a bleeding knee or a strained ankle. A place too, I realize, where everyone I ever meet will only know the dead-daughter me. Tom is one. Like Puck in *A Midsummer Night's Dream,* he's there one second, gone the next.

In the summer of 2010, five months after Rachel died, I fly to Ireland for a week-long walking retreat, a gift from some very generous friends.

Our group stops for lunch at a natural ridge protected from the earlier bleakness. A chain of shaggy brown sheep shuffle along beside us, oblivious to our presence. People huddle together and eat the sandwiches prepared for us that morning. I hold back, sit off to the side. Make plans.

In my black daypack are Rachel's ashes — enough to last me three weeks in Europe.

My attention is drawn toward a small rock pile. It reminds me of the balanced rock stacks that are common in Vancouver's Stanley Park. Built where land meets water, they require a sculptor's steady hand and a calm mind. This one will surely be gone by the end of the day. The winds on The Burren are fierce.

"Can I join you?" Tom sits down beside me, places his arm firmly around my back. I rest my head on his shoulder. A tremble.

"What do you think?" he says, pointing to the rock stack.

I nod.

"I made it."

"What?" I turn to face him. "Just now?"

"Yes, just now."

He pulls out a small blue book from inside his jacket.

"This is for you," he says, cupping the book in my palm.

I open it to the page he's marked. A poem titled "Rachel." Seeing her name in print makes my heart thump.

"Incredible. Where did you get this?"

"I found it. Yesterday. My first girlfriend was called Rachel, too."

How on Earth did he find this book? It was late afternoon when we'd arrived back into Ballyvaughan, a village with just a handful of shops. And it was just yesterday when we'd walked and talked together. When I'd told him about Rachel, he'd told me about his best friend's daughter. "She died last year from an asthma attack. She was only twenty-two."

One thing I know about grief is that if people know of yours, they'll more likely tell you of theirs. While some avoid the topic vehemently, or talk about frivolous things, perhaps hoping a "let's change the subject" strategy secures a distraction, Tom and I found refuge in the other.

I fumble with the zipper of my black daypack. Rachel's once. He sees me struggling.

"Do you need some help?"

I don't want to cry. But I start crying.

"I want to leave some of her ashes here."

I peel open the seal, poke my hand inside, take a huge pinch of her ashes, lean forward onto my knees and sprinkle her over the rock stack. Some of her ashes stick like a residue to my fingertips, so I wipe my hand on a tuft of grass, then sit back down beside Tom.

"She always wanted to come to Ireland."

He pulls me in tighter. We watch her ashes blow away.

Who did I tell about wanting to leave my daughter's ashes on my travels? My memory's unclear. Not my family, strangely. I thought they wouldn't understand. How could they when I didn't really know what I was doing either? But with Tom it was easy. And with Pascale.

In Zurich, Pascale had welcomed me to her country, calling out my name and waving through the glass doors, long before they opened into the crowd.

The next day she and I had cycled the forty kilometres around Lake Biel, cowbells clunking out their dull notes.

It's Rachel who's meant to be here. Not me. She and Pascale, my sister Sarah's homestay student, had met just once.

"Next time you go travelling," said Pascale, "you must come to Switzerland to see me."

"Thanks," Rachel had beamed. "I'd love to."

"Right here," Pascale called out. "Here!"

Turning to look back over my shoulder, there was Pascale, ebullient. Off her bike now, and pointing toward a church. Whitewashed walls, dark chocolate spire.

"I think Rachel would like it here," she nodded.

We sat side by side in a field of high green grasses, the tiny village of Sutz behind us, and rested our helmeted heads together. I'm comforted by her eagerness to find the best, most picturesque spot for a girl she met only once.

"And now, Rachel, you are in Switzerland." Her voice, like a proclamation, strong and melodic. As if with volume, Rachel might hear. As if.

Eighteen months had passed since Rachel died. It was the first time that someone called her name out loud.

I'd coerced my girlfriends to go with me. How they might "take it," watching me leave my daughter's ashes, I really had no idea. Just a hunch, that it was safe. Imperative.

The village of Bamburgh is located on England's Northumberland's coast. Four girls, three nights in a tiny stone cottage; it's our first time all together since we left high school over thirty years ago.

We are all mothers now. We understand love above everything else.

"I'm going to leave some of Rachel's ashes here."

We're standing on the pink golden sand of Embleton Bay. That's when I tell them. There's mixed feelings. One begins to cry. One freezes. One hugs me, "How fantastic. It'd be an honour."

I step away, roll up my jeans and untie my laces. The waves of the North Sea trickle in.

"I'll go out on my own. It's okay."

Turning back, I add a cautionary note. "I don't want you to be traumatized by her ashes flying off who knows where," chuckling like it's no big deal. They stand in a line, clasping each other's hands. I think they're relieved to keep a safe distance.

It's strange to be ankle deep in the ocean, knowing eyes are on your back. I hope my grief isn't a burden on my friends. I hope instead they'll go back home and show their children how much they're loved. Already I picture them pulling a son or daughter tight to their chest. Holding them longer than usual.

I lick my finger to test the wind, then throw a handful as far out as I can.

CHAPTER 6

NATURAL SWIMMER

Bunbury, in Western Australia, is a haven for dolphins. I see them all the time; it's an occurrence that eludes even the locals, I'm told. Not surprisingly, I start reading into things (my natural tendency). There's a feeling that Rachel might be among them, *is* one of them; that her death may not have been an end but rather a transformation.

It wouldn't be the first time. For months now Rachel has been tracking me. She was the white feather that landed at my feet on the afternoon I'd gone walking in Seattle, and the brittle leaf that drifted onto the table, beside the bottle of San Miguel, where I sat with my niece in Port de Pollença.

What you need to know is that Rachel was a natural swimmer, blessed with lithe, slender limbs and aquatic grace. She'd swum with dolphins in Kaikura, New Zealand, and joined the local *ragazzi* as they leapt from rocky outcrops into the warm Cinque Terre waters.

It wasn't always that way. I picture her as a newborn, a screaming baby in the tub above the sink, turning a deep purple as her body shivered in the warm water.

Like many impressionable preteens who watched the opening scene of *Free Willy*, Rachel dreamed of becoming a marine biologist. In her final summer, with chemotherapy treatment proving hugely successful, she pursued her childhood passion. Her first step was to volunteer at the Vancouver Aquarium. She researched available courses, made calls and readied a plan. I rarely saw her so energized. A good friend whose firm conviction that anything is possible effused nothing but praise for her tenacity and faith. I felt ashamed at the lack of mine. But like everything, we need to be ready. I wasn't. Rachel was.

"We have to be careful of the stories we tell about ourselves. There's nothing in a caterpillar that tells you it's going to be a butterfly," says Elisabet, an evolutionary biologist I'd met in Mallorca. "If it realized it were one and the same, it'd never change. Its transformation is so radical."

She recommends I read Stephanie Tolan's book, *Change Your Story, Change Your Life.*"

In Bunbury, I do.

In a home Bob and I bought together in North Vancouver, and with the immediate news of his terminal diagnosis, there were too few carefree memories. Bob and I were over before we began. Barely three years.

This memory, though, long after the architect left and our first dinner party was over, stays with me. Bob and I talked late into the night. The iPod was still playing, the dirty dishes still on the counter. We sat together at the kitchen table. He drew sketches on his pad of grid paper.

"I want to relocate the stairs over here... and the chimney I'll rebuild there, on the outside wall."

That was the plan.

Bob's favourite tune started to play. Jimmy Rogers All Stars, "Blow Wind Blow." He took my hand. Pulled me up. I didn't quite know how to move to the jazzy R&B rhythms. So I stepped back, watched as he raised his arms high above his head, dancing slowly, swaying his hips. God, I thought, what a dancer.

"Hey Beck," he said. "What d'ya think we'll be doing this time next year?"

I knew it even before I saw it. The break in the water. Slick grey, just metres from the beach. *She's swimming directly toward me.* The dolphin's body arcing up, then down.

My heart races and I don't know what to do. At first I freeze, not wanting to scare her away, but as she swims closer and closer I begin to walk toward her, my steps long and fast. Faster. So close now I want to run in fully clothed and touch her.

Might this be her world and mine coming together miles from where she left me? I want to believe it. I want to believe that Rachel has given over her human form, and is fluent now, in her own language. I want to believe she lives now in a different realm of being — in water, where one thing becomes another; a creature so gloriously fluid in its movement. Her young, agile body locked up like a prisoner is free at last and swimming again. No faltering. I want to believe she's called me here to witness her rebirth. And for that one moment, her life is intersecting with mine.

It must have been September, four months before she died, when she'd climbed out of the car at the Vancouver Aquarium and walked toward the Employees Only entrance. Her limp was getting worse. The foot brace hidden beneath her black Ecco boots did little to help. She turned around, waved goodbye and smiled. *See, Mum? I'm okay.*

I could follow her out to sea. But I don't. I watch her turn around and swim away.

Before leaving Vancouver I signed up to be a house-sitter, available to house-sit pretty much anywhere in the world. Flexibility was paramount to my having a place to sleep.

In late November 2011, during my final week in Mallorca, an email arrived.

This particular email alert, from House Carers, was for a month-long house-sit in Bunbury, Australia, a city two hours south of Perth. Already I missed the long days of summer, and I knew that far from England, Australia offered the promise of complete escape.

Surely nobody here would call on me to save a life.

Jacquie lives in Perth. An old friend, we'd almost lost touch. She picked up mid-ring, like she was standing by the phone waiting for my call.

"Hey, I landed a house-sit in Bunbury," I said. "I'm thinking I'll take it!"

"Fan-tastic," she says. "I'll be at the airport."

Three days later I'm on a plane to Zurich. To Singapore. To Perth.

And there it was, the first ripple of change.

There's solace in a shared past. This won't be the first time I mention this; trying to counterbalance how much misfortune a person can handle is a tricky business. That Jacquie had met Rachel, and knew about Bob, and had endured her own private grief, made my choice to come to Australia easier.

When my Bunbury house-sit finished, I move in with Jacquie for four weeks. The change of living situation is a panacea. In exchange for room and board, I cook. But that's not really all of it. It's much more. I hadn't known that I was starving for a deep sense of connection. Both of us knew what it was to suffer, and perhaps we helped the other suffer less.

I'd grown so used to my Mallorcan solitude, the elusiveness of my own secret club. Hearing myself talk. It sounded new. LOUD.

In 1997 Jacquie had joined the staff at our West Vancouver elementary school for a year's teaching exchange. Along with Bronwen, my teaching partner, the three of us became fast friends. In December 2001, Bronwen died of leukemia. She was thirty-four.

"I think about Bronwen all the time," says Jacquie, pulling out a wooden keepsake box as we sit on the carpet of her living room floor. I watch the contents spill out like a jack-in-the-box: emails, letters, cards, folded sheets of A4, all correspondence collected over the final weeks and months of Bronwen's life. Ten years ago exactly. Jacquie dips into the box, unfolding each item, then reading out loud. She probably hasn't done this in years. I notice the sad weight in her face.

Grief by its very nature is a lonely time. But for Jacquie, so far away from Canada, it was especially lonely.

"You had each other, but this was all I had."

The sky in Perth is blue. It's always blue. Hot bright blue.

On these sharpened sunny days I stop at the tree where the ravens congregate. Their communal sigh, a slow, lingering *ah-ah-aaaah,* merges with the warm currents above the Indian Ocean. As if freedom were the greatest gift of every living thing. Detecting an open path ahead, I mimic their sigh.

This feeling is new. I'd never liked crows. Not Canadian crows. There were always too many around our home. Bob's and my new home. Springtime the air was black with crows.

Then the chickadees came.

It's an amazing sight to watch birds making a nest. It takes weeks. But Bob and I had the time. These were the early days after his diagnosis, and I had taken a leave from my teaching job.

It was a sunny May day when the chickadees left. I hardly noticed the first one squeeze out from the tiny opening, or the second. The others struggled. Some fell from the kitchen window ledge, unaware of the grasp at their feet. Two hid behind my pot of rosemary. One smashed into the kitchen window, stunned. I ran inside to fetch the soft broom, gently brushed it on its way. Eventually the nest was empty. Nothing else came out. It all happened so quickly. An hour, at most. Bob missed it. He was sleeping more and more.

"To be expected," said the doctor.

For the next three years Rachel and I watched the annual exodus together. One year I wish we hadn't. A crow snatched a fledgling, flew onto the roof of our garage and ate it. We watched it ripping flesh from bone, unable to look away. All that care come to nothing.

Four months after Rachel died I put the house up for sale. Before the first Open House, I caught sight of a tiny chickadee stuck on the deck.

I had a plan. With the front door wedged open, I headed back to the deck, cupped the chickadee in my hands. I felt its panicked wings against my palms, its wild heart banging into the dark cavity.

"It's okay, buddy, I gotcha."

I speed walked out to the front yard, my arms outstretched; it didn't see my face screwed up, "ew-ew-ew," a live bird in my hands.

The hydrangea bush beneath the living room window is where I left it. I opened my palms near the dirt. It just stood there. But I never returned to check its fate. There's a limit to how much a parent can do to save their child. I know this now.

CHAPTER 7

LIMPS TO STUMBLES

Nothing prepares you. Not logic nor time nor doctors.

It is October 16, 2009. Daryl's sixtieth birthday. This day marks the beginning of the end of her life.

Daryl, my ex-husband, Rachel's father, scrambles into the back seat outside the Hotel Vancouver, our usual pickup spot en route to the Cancer Agency.

"Happy Birthday," I say, as he slams the door.

"Happy Birthday, Dad," Rachel turns to him and smiles.

"Thanks, babe."

It would be a long winter of white skies. We gather together in a tiny overlit room: Rachel, Daryl and I, Dr. Theissen and his nurse, Roslyn, just as we've been doing for years now. Almost eight. The usual tests have been conducted. The medications, they confirm, are no longer working. And the room is silent.

"Is this going to kill me?"

They nod.

Rachel's face. Just seconds after. Bright eyed and smiling. Waiting to see my reaction? It's hard to tell if the news confirms what she'd suspected, or if it's a hideous shock.

None of us cry.

She links her arm in mine as we walk back to the parking lot.

Sometimes the best we have is denial. Despite all the evidence, the seizure at fifteen, two craniotomies, the radiation, the needles, the chemotherapy, the dire statistics on brain tumour survival rates, and now the limping, we denied it all.

I tried. Maybe she did too. If so, I don't remember. Rachel wasn't the "let's talk about feelings" kind. The interpretive musings of metaphor and meaning that her sister Charlotte craved, and I indulged, Rachel found trite.

"Can't we just enjoy the movie?" she'd say.

To pursue the difficult conversation felt more about me, and my needs.

We didn't talk about it. Then we couldn't. She could barely speak.

Bob and I had talked constantly. But at forty-eight, he accepted that an early death was to be his. Seven months and long hours of courageous conversation helped us both reconcile his death, and my grief at his leaving.

And even if Rachel and I had talked, what did I expect to hear? "Sure, Mum. I'm okay with dying at twenty-three."

A young adult willingly relinquishing life seems implausible. But that day when Roger Daltrey was blasting from the Bose, "My Generation," we sang along. I'd forgotten that line until it was almost upon us. Suddenly I ached for the song to stop. But it didn't. Instead we caught ourselves staring at the other and singing, "Hope I die before I get old." Her eyes swollen and glassy as if to say, "I get it, Mum. It's okay."

How many words does an adult speak in an average day? Google suggests for women, somewhere in the range of five to twenty thousand. With trouble in the brain, you're reduced to essentials. Word choice demands an acuity most of us can't envisage. It's folly to assume we'll never run out of words.

Only three months earlier I'd opened the back door, walked into the kitchen and watched as she unloaded the dishwasher. With her left hand. Her right arm, dead at her side.

"Hi, Mum."

She talked about her day. It was a struggle to follow. Still, I hung on to every word. Before they were blanketed with silence. How many more times would she call my name?

"It's to be expected," said Dr. Theissen. "As the swelling increases she'll lose the ability to understand letters and words. She'll know what she wants to say, but be unable to say it."

"Will she understand what I say to *her*?"

"Sadly, no. Toward the end you'll be unable to communicate with her. With this kind of tumour all language capabilities are lost. I'm so sorry."

"How about sign language? Blinking? Pictures?" I caught my breath. "Surely there must be some way I can let my daughter know how much I..."

He turned his head from side to side.

But he wasn't done.

"You'll need to move her bedroom upstairs."

I head down to Rachel's bedroom, the room she's made for herself. Tidy, but not clean.

A world map consumes most of one wall. A poster of Orlando Bloom as Legolas, on another. Beneath the window, a wicker basket of stuffed toys from her first surgery gathers dust.

A Chinese egg in a glass case, a gift from her friend Katherine: "Rachel was the first person to welcome me when I arrived from Hong Kong." Beside it, a miniature blue car plate, RACHEL in raised white letters, a souvenir from Universal Studios. She's there now. Ten days in California with her dad.

Boarding passes, concert ticket stubs and photo booth strips of crazy faces are pinned neatly within the borders of the wood frame of a corkboard. There are dusty candles she never burns, curtains she rarely opens. On her desk, the black bristles of her coiled brush are heavy with hair, and I wonder if she ever thinks to clean it out. I run my finger through the dust on her bedside table.

Her clothes organized on the Home Depot shelves: sleeveless tops at one end, jackets at the other. The dark woven basket on the top shelf is where I know she keeps her scarves, each one folded neatly.

My friend Cathy calls down the stairwell. "The guys are here to move her bed."

"Okay." But I doubt she heard me. She's talking, offering them a cup of tea.

I'm sitting on her bed now. Her fleece blanket is covered with stars and our rescue dog Jack's fur. There's Scruffy on her pillow, her long time stuffy, his cappuccino coat all matted, like he got wet and never dried properly. How long had she had him now? A decade at least. She'd brought him to Australia when we'd lived there, a year by the beach.

"Where do you want the bookcase to go?" Cathy calls out.

I call back to her, up the stairs. "You do it, Cath. I can't think anymore."

I pack the small stuff into a box. Stuff I figure she'd like in her new bedroom — her two travel scrapbooks, the corkboard, some DVDs — a kind of anthology of her loves and travels. She'd call it a menagerie. It was her favourite word, the way it sounded out loud. Or was it plethora?

A brain tumour is a slow, methodical killer. It destroys body parts in progression. Strides turn to steps. Limps to stumbles. Numbness to dead weight.

The phone rang on the day she climbed Mount Ngauruhoe in New Zealand. Bob answered. They chatted briefly.

"Yup, she's right here. Hold on." My hand was already reaching out for the receiver.

"Mum, best hike of my life."

It was a great connection, as if she were calling from next door.

"I looked down on the clouds," she said. "The Red Crater was amazing; the valleys were all steaming patches of rock and earth, like a Martian landscape."

I'd never heard her like this. So overjoyed.

"It took us nine hours. I've looked at my photos but they don't really capture the view."

"Nine hours!"

"Yeah. Mount Doom in *Lord of the Rings*."

"Brilliant."

Two years later, summer 2007, she walked the coastal path of Italy's Cinque Terra. At each town, swam in the sea.

Four months before she died she could still walk to the bus stop.

Up the garden path. Down the garden path.

I forget when she could still walk from her bedroom to the bathroom.

By October's end she limped, leaning on walls or the shoulders of whoever was around. Early in December she was bed-ridden. It all happened so quickly, her fading from fullness. To watch the awkward gait, the painstaking effort of consecutive steps was heart wrenching. How did it feel for her? As we watched?

Daryl bought a wheelchair. She hated it.

It's a soggy November morning, a thick damp sky, when I drive us across town to Granville Island. She's wearing her brown American Eagle blazer. A chunky pink scarf is wrapped twice at her neck, and a funky knitted toque purchased from a street vendor in New York is pulled down over her ears. She looks gorgeous. But the wheelchair, like a lightning rod, draws stares from the market goers.

It was a very short trip.

I pile the wheelchair into the back seat, then lower Rachel into the front. The weather can't make up its mind. I'm over-dressed, sweating under the layers.

The clerk puts down the phone as I wrestle with the door, rushes over to hold it open.

"Kerry will be with you in just a moment."

We wait in the silent office, just the hum of fluorescent ceiling lights.

"Hi, Rachel. How're you doing today?" Kerry is a Notary Public with shoulder-length blonde hair and big eyes. Her suit jacket is buttoned at the waist, a great look for a full-breasted woman.

"I gather you're here to authorize your mum as your Power of Attorney. Is that right?"

Rachel nods.

The secretary holds a pile of papers, tapping it on the desk to align the edges perfectly, then hands it to Kerry. The women mumble something. Nod.

"Does it matter which hand she uses to sign her name?" I ask.

"Whichever hand she's used all this time," says Kerry. "That's the hand she should use."

Her right hand, then, the one she used to write her first words. RNBW, FMY, UNCN in blue Crayola jumbo felts.

Rachel reaches for the pen.

I lift it, put it in her hand. She squeezes the wrist of her right hand with her left. I put my hand over top, to steady the pen.

"*Please*, let her do this on her own," Kerry says. "This is a legal document."

So I hold the sheet still.

We watch as the writing of a preschooler appears. Watch her strain to make it resemble something like her name. The black line is left empty, stranded on the page. Of all the indignities in her dying, this was high on the list. If Rachel apologized I don't remember. But there it was for all of us to see. For her to see.

I want to tell the nice woman about Rachel's writing: how she drew a circle for the dot over "i" and made the letter "a" like a typewriter. I want to make explicit how she'd written her favourite recipes in my ancient cookbook; her letters full of energy, bold on the page, like art.

Back in the waiting room, we sit together in silence. Aching tightness in my throat. *Don't cry. Please don't cry. She hates it when you cry.*

"Here you go," says the young assistant, balancing on her stilettos. She hands me the envelope.

"Thank you." My voice is all wobbly. Rachel looks at me. It isn't a look I've seen before. Something like disgust.

Later that month Daryl takes her to California. In preparation she and I shop for a bra. Nothing works.

"Try this one," says the sales assistant, "it has the easiest clasp."

She had no idea. But why would she? It's unlikely you'd recognize a brain tumour patient. There are no wraithlike features typical of many cancer patients. It's only toward the end, with the heavy use of steroids, that the swollen face might give them away. Plumped up, cherub-like, almost glowing.

Rachel begins to cry, throwing them all onto the floor. Not so much weeping but a full on outburst. Noisy. Messy. Suddenly I'm hit by a surge of indescribable sorrow. Rachel didn't do anger. It was tragic, and yet a great relief.

At Disneyland, Daryl wheels her to the front of every line. In Arizona, they take a helicopter tour of the Grand Canyon. In Vegas, a glider ride over the desert.

Michael Henderson, a pilot at the Soaring Centre in Jean, Nevada, has seen many who've had a glider ride on their to-do list. An email he sent to Daryl after that ride read:

> We've had our share of some six thousand people at the glider centre. Rachel was different. More sensitive. Once we were up in the air I could see her staring at the ground. She seemed fixed on something.
> "I see a plane down there," she said. "It seems to have a wing missing."
> "Yes, it's broken," I said. "We're working to get it fixed."
> She was silent for a while.
> "Just like me."
> I choked up. To someone who's flown all kinds of folks for forty-two years, I can't explain, even now, how cool, even poetic that still is.

Two men carry a hospital bed in through the front door as Andy Williams sings, "It's-the-most, won-der-ful-time-of-the-year."

Rachel hides. Lays down her head on the sofa, pulls the tasselled throw over her face. Charlotte helps.

Days later a crimson metal box is dropped off at the house while I'm at work. It looks like a giant toolbox except it's full of needles and medicines. It takes up most of the kitchen counter. We don't touch it. It's only for the nurses.

Inside the fridge is a bunch of clear plastic syringes wedged inside a pale green tumbler, like headless flowers vying for space in too small a vase. They're loaded up with liquids. A nurse comes over. She shows us how to connect the ends to the plastic flaps hanging from Rachel's body: two in one arm, one in the other, and one in her dead leg. Daryl sticks a sheet of plain paper to the kitchen counter. On it are the dosages and times of day and night we have to pump our daughter's veins.

Days later they bring the commode.

On top of the fridge is a three-ring black binder.

"What's this?" I ask the doctor.

She pulls it down, unclicks the metal and passes me a sheet, Do Not Resuscitate emblazoned across the top.

"You have to sign this," she says.

"Why?"

"It gives authorization for no medical interference to be provided for Rachel…because…she's a terminal patient."

She hands me a black pen.

On Boxing Day, the palliative nurse sits us down in the kitchen, announces her news. "A bed's come free on the palliative ward. We think Rachel should take it. Let me know as soon as you can."

Daryl and I creep into her room. We've piled her Christmas presents beneath the only clothes she wears — three tank tops, hanging on a rod. One is a ribbed pale grey; one, a salmon colour; and the other is burgundy with squiggles of silver thread running through. All from American Eagle, her favourite store.

All those years, offering up two options: Cheese or pepperoni? Cheerios or Weetabix? This jacket or that coat? And now, I have to ask her this one.

I've spent weeks now, choosing my words meticulously so that a nod or a single word might be enough. Not easy for someone who talks so much. Like a new mother with a two-year-old, it means honing in on what really matters.

"Where do you want to…?"

"Would you rather be in hospital or at home until…?"

"The nurse thinks you should take it, Rach. What do you think?"

A mother can't carry this question alone. We wait, Daryl and I, probing her face, her lips. Her cocoa eyes robbed of all but her gentle soul, glisten in the winter light of her makeshift bedroom.

"Home," she says.

"You sure?"

"Mmm," and she smiles. "Home."

I walk away, pick up the phone on the kitchen counter, strangle a cry.

"You can give the room to someone else."

Then I run the tap, wash the wine glasses. I want to cry but I can't. I want to slide to the floor, clutch my belly and wail, but I can't do that either. I want to go back to bed and scream into the pillows but she is in the room next to mine. Besides, what is the big deal? She'd just told me the truth. So, I don't cry. She might think I'd wished for a different answer, or that her dad and I were so exhausted, needed to sleep.

Daryl shakes his head, "Hold it together, Beck. You're not the one that's dying."

You may think that living with a brain tumour since age fifteen meant her lifestyle would've been compromised. You'd be wrong. Only in the final four months of her life did her body fail her.

We're a family of dancers. Great dancers. Every celebration ends with dancing. We crank the music and take to the floor. Thanksgiving had been no different, except for one thing: Rachel's arm, the dead weight of her right arm, hanging limp at her side. You'd have been blind not to notice. Look at her face, and nothing had changed: her trademark smile, her shiny eyes.

None of us mentioned it. Not until the next day at breakfast.

"When did she get so bad?" Charlotte said. "Am I the only one who didn't know this?" Questions that can't be answered quickly, or easily. Not in this fixer-upper house with no soundproofing, where every step is a creak and every whisper overheard.

How, exactly, do you tell your younger daughter that her older sister is dying? When denial is the best way to sidestep the truth?

And then it's New Year's Eve. Rachel watches from her hospital bed, Charlotte and I singing together. Dancing like it was closing night, our final performance, a spectacular send-off for what we all know will be our last together. All of us, lawbreakers of the no-longer-a-secret, secret.

The song "I Gotta Feeling" by The Black Eyed Peas, Rachel's favourite, blasting now so loudly I have to touch the glass in the coffee table to stop it vibrating.

We turn to look at Rachel. God knows why. I thought it was the cruelest thing we could have done, flaunting our agility like that. Her hospital bed, we'd aligned perfectly so she could see the action in the living room.

Beneath the layers of morphine she opens her eyes. Smiles.

I yell in Charlotte's ear, my hands cupped like parentheses.

"This feels awful."

"Don't worry, Mum," her eyes locked on mine, "she wouldn't want it any other way."

Again, I peek over at Rachel. Just for a second. There she is, her full face looking back at me. Watching. Watching. She raises her hospital bed to get a better view.

We sing louder. So loud that our voices sound more like cries.

It's early January 2010. I'm on an indefinite leave from my teaching job.

"I'm not going back to work," I say, and she starts to cry. She'd cried a week earlier, too, when Daryl had moved into her old bedroom in the basement.

I pull down the book *Unforgettable Places to See Before You Die* from the shelf, and I lay down beside Rachel.

"Do you want to look at this?"

She nods. Her cheeks are flushed and swollen from the flood of steroids in her failing body. Her speech, almost gone.

The title felt barbaric, as if I was tipping her off on what would surely be her fate: dying young. But in 2007 I bought the book anyway. In it were places she'd already seen, and I liked that.

The pages still smell new. In blue pen she's drawn stars, five-pointed stars, beside the Grand Canyon, The Alhambra, Chichén Itzá, Venice, Manhattan, Santorini, Uluru, the Great Barrier Reef. I turn the pages quickly of those she'll miss: Ankor Wat, Zanzibar, St. Petersburg.

When I get to the Taj Mahal I stop, look at her.

"One day I'm going there," she'd said, opening the book that Christmas morning.

"Are you okay with this?"

She smiles.

Rachel's long brown curls become a burden for the caregivers. I hear her groan when they turn her. Loose strands pulled beneath the weight of her head. Daryl phones around, tells them our predicament. A lady volunteers her time. She lays the scissors on the kitchen table, the best place to do the cutting. "She tied you to a kitchen chair." So goes the Leonard Cohen lyric of "Hallelujah."

Does she look out onto the deck, cold and empty on that January morning? Or is it just her reflection she sees smacked up against the glass?

"I know this room. I've walked this floor."

What, I wonder, does she remember? The small gathering after Bob died? The chickadee's struggle for freedom? The jigsaw puzzle, Country Dog Gentlemen, extending beyond the edges of the patio table? How we'd made a frame of the straight-edged pieces, a framework in which to safely dabble with the rest. Does she remember how we wilted beneath the fiberglass roof in the summer heat? Or the time Jack snatched our sushi as we ran inside for chopsticks?

Worst of all, does she look to the back gate, to the path she'd walked so often? To an old life that stretched out before her, now gone. Does she watch as her hair falls onto the hardwood floor? Or does she keep her eyes closed?

Say goodbye to the long hair, I thought. Get used to saying goodbye.

I leave before the cutting begins.

"Don't cut it too short."

Jack races out as I roll in, back from a walk in the woods. Rachel is searching for a better look in the window's reflection, her left hand grasping for something at her neck, not there.

Rachel had a face that could carry short hair: big brown eyes that framed her high cheekbones, a clear complexion, an enviably cute nose and thick, luscious lips. When she smiled, as she so often did, there was just more of her to love. At fourteen, she'd modelled for Toni and Guy. We'd watched on *Breakfast Television* as the stylists ran their fingers through her fine hair; heavy highlights and choppy ends were this season's fashion.

There must have been hair on the floor, but I don't remember seeing any. Daryl, fastidious, is sweeping up with my red broom.

There would be no more fixing her hair for a Saturday night out or rifling through her clothes for the outfit she'd eventually wear for a night in the city.

Her father, the pragmatist, thought it practical and perfect.

"Looks great, kiddo. Much better for everyone."

Suggesting it'll grow is pointless. We're counting the days.

At fifteen, approaching her first brain surgery, it was her one question. Would they have to cut her hair, or worse still, shave her head?

"You don't have to like it," said the neurosurgeon. "But here's the facts."

I braced myself against the arms of the chair, just as I had years ago waiting in the front car of Space Mountain, the brand-new ride at Disneyland. When the bar was lowered there would be no going back.

"We'll be strapping you to the table."

He fixed his eyes on Rachel.

"To access your brain we need to remove a large portion of your skull."

He drew an imaginary line, pushing down his thick white hair to show the C-shaped drill line they had planned for her.

"It's called an awake craniotomy. We need you to talk to us while we operate."

Did I hold Rachel's hand or was she beyond that now?

She'd chosen the surgery. The surgeon's "watch and wait" option was not for her. She needed to know what was really in her head. Who wouldn't at her age?

"We'll be using staples, not stitches, to close it all back to-gether. You might like to keep them. Show them to your friends." He brushed his hands together like one does to remove flour from their fingers.

"Don't worry, you won't feel a thing."

The image of a staple gun against my daughter's head, the sound burst of metal shooting into bone, revolted me. When I tell this story to friends in the staff room, one tells me later she excused herself to go to the bathroom to cry.

With my daughters so young, I'd expected some gentleness from this man. Rachel was fifteen, Charlotte thirteen. But to him, it didn't seem to matter. We'd need to toughen up.

Her surgery was the first awake craniotomy performed at BC Children's Hospital. It would be videotaped; interns and residents would watch from the gallery above the operating table.

She asked about her hair.

"Yes," he said, leaning back, hands behind his head, "you can keep that lovely long hair. We'll just trim it along the incision line." His thumb and index finger showed us just how much. Almost an inch.

Rachel and I exchanged glances, but nothing about her face was telling. I had no idea how she felt.

He leaned sideways to look at Charlotte and Daryl.

"You two okay back there?"

His fingertips, I remember, pressed hard into the oak desk, turning white.

I turned to look behind me. Daryl, rocking forward and back, elbows on his knees, carried his head in his hands. His bald spot had grown since our divorce; his fine, blond hair had disappeared entirely from the crown. It exposed the shiny pink of scalp. Charlotte was bent over, close to fainting.

"Just a bit dizzy," said Charlotte, to the air between her calves. Ribbons of her bleach-streaked hair brushed the floor, swinging left, then right.

I take the SeaBus downtown. The sky is bright and there's a dry chill. Bundled in my favourite gabardine trench coat, chocolate brown with buttons of brushed gold, I head off on a thrilling adventure. I even wear makeup.

Later that afternoon when the light has faded, I tiptoe into Rachel's bedroom. She opens her eyes. Smiles.

"You like it?"

She nods.

My hair looked great. We both knew it. Utilitarian would best describe hers.

I should have walked out right then. Carolynne was Rachel's discovery. Why I couldn't have taken my chance on a stylist close to home I still don't understand. It was cruel how I pointed to Carolynne's business card pinned to the corkboard on the wall at the end of her bed.

"I went to Colourbox too," I say. "Carolynne says Hi."

I lift Jack onto her bed. He leaps away before Rachel can touch him.

A skittish dog, he never stayed long. Not now. A slight adjustment of her hospital bed and he was gone. When she was downstairs in her old bedroom, he'd slept every night at the foot of her bed. Same blue and green Ikea duvet cover, same fleece blanket, but everything else had changed.

Up in the Air had just been released. It was playing at the Fifth Avenue cinemas in Kitsilano. A long way, except it wasn't. Only that my world had radically shrunk by ever-increasing degrees.

She's sleeping when I leave.

Me. Alone. Watching a movie.

This was nothing so shocking. For the past two years I'd often put my needs before hers. Peter, a former boyfriend, and I had run into each other fourteen months after Bob died, dated ever since. Chemotherapy, her white blood cell count sometimes dangerously low, didn't change things.

"Peter's coming over for dinner, staying the night."

She never complained. Perhaps she understood, too, that the time I spent with Peter was what made those final months bearable.

I drive off on the lit streets of North Vancouver, hands gripped at 10 and 2 on the steering wheel. The seat, hard at my back. The route I'd practised in my mind earlier that evening. Nothing could jeopardize my return. Backing out the carport I hit the upturned garbage bin. *Shit.* Slamming the car door a second time might wake her. She'll know I've left.

I'm crossing over the Lions Gate Bridge when the panic hits. The car was moving at eighty kilometres per hour with me in it. So fast. Rachel so far away.

Hardly a moment later, I am driving in downtown Vancouver. The city lights, the traffic lights, people crossing crosswalks, hands in pockets, puffy jackets zipped to the chin, and me accelerating on. *My daughter is dying and I'm going to see a movie.*

Back at home I underplay my enthusiasm about how much I'd enjoyed the chemistry between Clooney and his costar.

I'd asked for extra butter on my popcorn, washed my hands thoroughly before entering her room. That smell. It would have felt like rubbing salt in a wound.

Just days later Rachel wakes from a long nap, whispers something. I can't be sure exactly what. The air moves through her lips, vibrating out as a word. It sounds like "Hospital."

"You want to go to the hospital?"

Daryl and I stare into her eyes. She nods.

It's coming close, she knows it.

Is that enough? A nod? You have to be certain. You can't mess this up. Not like all the other times in the years of parenting.

"You sure?"

A nod.

I watch myself pick up the phone, my yellow reflection moving through the lit kitchen against the pitch-black night.

"Seven West," the nurse says.

"Is a room ready?"

"Yes."

"Give us an hour," I say.

Not ten minutes later there's a knock at the front door. There's an ambulance outside. A fire truck behind it. Men in dark clothes forge their way in.

"This way," says Daryl.

Plate in one hand, fork in the other, I poke my head inside her bedroom.

Lined up along three sides, dark shapes lean in to execute the loading operation. I notice the badges sewn on the sleeve of their dark blue uniform. The room small, the men take up most of it.

Leaning back against the bathroom door, I shovel in some food, the front door still wide open. No tearing wind or thrashing rain, nothing dangerous or wet. A calm night, a crisp winter chill. I shiver. Men are coming back out. Better get out of the way.

The hall light illuminates the front steps. Men are talking loudly. The back doors of the ambulance open from the inside. A flurry of bodies works in unison. They drive off in the dark. I close the front door.

What the hell just happened?

They must have taken my daughter.

Back in the kitchen, I ask Daryl, "What would she like in the hospital? What should we take?"

We shove down a couple more bites of the cold chicken then slip the plates into the sink.

"I suppose we leave the syringes in the fridge."

I walk back into her bedroom.

A chunk of beige synthetic blanket is pooled at the foot of the bed. A mass of sheeting yanked away from its moorings is dragging on the floor. The room is absolutely silent.

Why did she change her mind? Why hospital?

Jack sniffs the front door. He runs down to the basement, back up again, racing into her room, then over to me. I watch him from behind the kitchen counter, then pick up the receiver. The same nurse answers, "Seven West."

"She's on her way."

I look into his nervous brown eyes, scratching behind his ears until he calms. "It's okay, I'll be back later."

On top of the fridge is the black binder. There was no need for that now.

For three days we take shifts back to the house.

Climb the steps.

Open the door.

Feed the dog.

Walk the dog.

Check for messages.

Lock the door.

Walk.

Six blocks.

Watching.

Waiting.

One day I arrive home and her hospital bed has gone. There are dust balls on her bedroom floor, some dried-up Kleenex. The diapers are still stacked on the bookshelf. The fish lurch in the tank. The gaudy lit fluorescent pinks and yellows. I notice now.

I sit on the hardwood floor, resting my back against the cold plaster, and look through an old photograph album. The toddler in the turban, the fine crocheted baby blue scarf holding up the ringlets, knotted at the front, my favourite. She doesn't know the picture is being taken. Another in Lake Mackenzie on Fraser Island, posing for the camera in her white-trimmed black bikini, her arms flung wide, the length of her modelling legs magnified in the crystal blue water. A timeless image of youth and youthful promise.

At twelve years old, she was already middle-aged and none of us knew it. There was nothing in this photo that said she would end her days unable to move or speak.

Her graduation photo sits framed on another shelf. Hard to know what to look at first. A scream of hot pink and sparkling hair clips, or the smile — an event in itself that said, "I did it." The stylist had swept her short hair into an updo just as she'd wanted. Nobody would've known there was a brain tumour in there.

I pull the photos out and leave them on the shelf. Already we're gathering favourites for the slide show.

Jack cocks his head, looks at me confused.

"She's not coming back."

Rachel was the kind of girl who loved an adventure. Years ago, living in Australia, we'd borrowed bikes from Daintree Crocodylus Youth Hostel, ridden north.

Giant ferns as tall as houses lined the roadside. We stopped at a tea plantation where they sold ice cream. We both opted for the four-scoop special: Soursop, Wattleseed, Black Sapote, and Macadamia Nut, and sat together on resin chairs at a chipped metal table, the melting drops hitting the dried dirt between our sandals. The seller had a bowl of each fruit out on display. The Soursop was a green, spikey orb; the Black Sapote, she said, was used for making chocolate pudding; and the Wattleseed tasted like coffee.

It was just the two of us on that day. Our easy companionship, our shared appreciation, living on the other side of the globe, letting the world of Australia change us. I loved that.

Pedalling home through thick jungle, we caught a flash of kingfisher blue. Rachel saw it first, braked hard.

"MUM! Stop." A tall bird, with a splash of red against a luminescent blue neck, stood frozen.

"I think it's a cassowary," she whispered.

Everything was still. I could hear the sound of my breath, my heart beating. And then off it went, dashing into the darkness like a dinosaur bouncing through the undergrowth. Then we lost sight of it.

In the hospital room, Daryl and I sit on chairs, our bodies angled at the hip, our faces inches from Rachel's. Almost touching. It's almost time.

"Natalie's on her way home," says Daryl. "She's on a plane right now."

"Is there anything you'd like to say to her?" I ask, "If she were here?"

Rachel's silent, straining for words for her best friend. I want to squeeze out every last one, push her brain to its limits.

"Follow your heart."

Daryl and I turn to each other. Disbelief, not because of the clarity and conviction of her words, or because the doctors were wrong — she could, in fact, communicate with us right till the very end — but because I'd never have pegged Rachel with these words. Clichéd like some billboard at Valentine's.

"How about Mum and I take your ashes whenever we go away?"

She nods. Yes.

"Keep you travelling?"

Nods again.

Our plans to cremate her body; an appalling admission.

Howard Shore's "Twilight and Shadow" plays on the small CD player beside her bed. Everything else falls away. I want to imagine she pictures herself like Frodo stepping into the boat, a Gandalphian wizard holding out his hand to guide her in, and together, them sailing off to white shores. Her Eden.

I know this is just how it should be, her dying this way, the poignant melodies calming her final hours. Tending to her senses for the passage ahead. But I may have been imagining too much. Perhaps a plane crash would have been her choice. At least she'd have been dying in motion.

Daryl says one last thing: "You're cleared for takeoff."

It's just after 4 a.m. when the nurse wakes us, flooding the room with fluorescent light. And I know then, we'd missed her final breaths. If she'd struggled I'd have never known. She'd waited till we were all asleep to slip away.

"People die the way they live," the doctor had said. "I see it every time."

The nurse brings us tea in bone china cups and saucers. They're covered in roses, rimmed with gold, just like my grandma's Royal Albert. Protocol, I thought, to ease us over the cliff edge — how many others had drunk from these cups — and yet strangely comforting. I thought of my mother. In Britain, a cup of tea is the perfect salve. "Let's put the kettle on. Have a cup of tea." She would have done the same thing, even the same 'Nice' biscuit in the saucer.

Around 5 a.m. Daryl picks up the box of leftover pizza, then heads out.

"Her energy's back in the universe," he says. "She isn't here anymore." He drives across the city raging at a hundred kilometres an hour. You can do that in the early morning hours when the lights flash green.

It's five, and now it's six. The room is silent and warm. Dark and warm. Just warm enough in my T-shirt, my socks on the linoleum. That cozy warmth of a dimmed table lamp is the only light. There's a covered fluorescent rod affixed to the wall above her bed but it's been turned off. Her face is calm. That raging red swelling is gone. Lying there under the pale-coloured blankets, the white sheets, all crinkled, she's so still. I slump forward, stare at her fingers, her long fingers and long nails, at the perfect square adhesive patch that holds a needle to the back of her hand.

I am alone now. Daryl has been gone for a while, and the nurses collected my teacup and saucer a long time ago. I drank the tea, all of it, without spilling, only crumbs from the biscuit in the saucer. Outside the dark is lifting for another dark, the first signs of morning. When's it time? You never know if it's too soon, or if it's too late. With Bob I'd stayed seven hours. Climbed in beside him, my hand on his chest, not moving. The nurse had brought in hot blankets and tucked them in around us. His blood pooled purple where his skin touched the sheets.

But this is different. If I don't go now I might never leave.

I have to leave in the darkness.

I have to walk home.

I have to go. Now.

The first light of day is brightening the skies.

But how can I leave?

One time, I almost make it to the door.

If I don't go now I think I never will.

I rock back and forth for momentum.

I'm standing.

I'm leaning over her bed, peeling away the pale pink blanket I knitted before her first surgery, wrapping it around my shoulders. The static sticks to my fleece; the crackle shocks me a little.

Careful not to wake her, I lift Scruffy from her pillow and wedge him under my arm. I bend down and kiss her cheek one last time. Another, on her forehead. Did I pull the covers up to her neck? My throat aches. A hard, swelling lump.

Inhale.

Just one breath.

The best you can do.

The deepest of your life.

Head for the door.

Don't look back. Not again.

Turn right.

You can do it.

Hold it in.

Until you're outside. In the fresh air.

A tugging backward.

Walk faster.

Almost there.

The corridor, an impassable sea.

Pass the nurses' station.

Hands on the double doors now.

Wire mesh in the glass.

Push.

The top of the stairs.

Another door.

Seven flights down.

Almost there.

"Come back!" A nurse rushes out. "We need you a moment."

What?

"Could you sign this?"

Furious scribbling. Blind.

Turn again for the doors.

"Hold on," the nurse grabs your hand. "Wait a second. We have some of Rachel's things."

She makes you wait.

Don't look back.

Wriggle.

Don't look. Not down that corridor.

There's only so much breath.

She slides over a small saucer, touches the back of your hand. "I'm so sorry."

Don't look up.

Snatch them up in your palm.

No memory. Still none.

"We took these from her when she came in last Tuesday."

The ring. The Celtic ring. Did I put it on?

She slides over a sheet of paper, points to where I should sign.
Done.
Down.
Turn.
Down.
Turn.
Not too fast.
Don't trip.
Polished linoleum.
Beige.
The giant mural. Garish.
Welcome to the World.
Three more flights.
There they are.
Double doors.
Opening. Too slow. T-o-o s-l-o-w.
Why didn't they feel me coming?
Run.
Sidewalk.
Stop.
Burst.

The icy January air shocked me. I pulled her blanket tight to my neck, bundling my ears and chin in the folds. Still warm. I drew Scruffy to my chest. His eyes, looking up at me. His nose, just a few black stitches, from all that loving. My free hand, a fist in my fleece pocket, I pulled tight around my belly to keep out the sharp cold.

What do I do now?

I looked down at my feet. My feet touched the sidewalk, again and again. I watched the laces moving at the end of the loops.

Keep walking. Don't stop.

I remembered trading hands, passing Scruffy into my warm hand, then plunging my frozen hand into the other pocket so tight I thought the seam might break and my fist might come lose. My eyes were streaming from the shock. My nose too. I swiped my sleeve upward across my face to absorb the drip. There was a hard, balled-up Kleenex in one pocket. It made things worse. It scratched the soft skin at the outer edges of my eyes.

There were few cars on the road on that Sunday morning. A passing driver might have noticed a woman with her head down, watching her every step. They would not have known the effort it required, or how each step separated her world from her daughter's. That even though it was inevitable, she wasn't ready for that separation. Prepared is not the same as ready. They wouldn't have known she was walking home in a frozen world from the same hospital where her daughter had been born twenty-three years earlier, and who died moments earlier. They wouldn't have noticed her lips mouthing, "Right. Left. Right."

They wouldn't have known the reason for her snail-like pace, or seen the invisible wire pulling her home, wrenching her back, like a pulley. Both, equally possible. They would never have known anything had changed so profoundly. But everything had.

They wouldn't know she was on the mission of a lifetime.

Then came the corner, the sharp turn left onto a new street. My feet turned. I know because I watched them. They followed the sidewalk, heading north. I wanted to keep going forever, to never stop. Maybe I could walk across the world. Never stopping.

My focus settled on the rhythm of my steps. It was about then when I discovered that I was not alone. As if I were a puppeteer pulling at strings. Two pairs of legs were walking me home: mine and not mine. One guiding the other. *Whose were the others?*

I passed the playground where my daughters spent half their childhood, but I didn't look up to see the swings or the slide or the roundabout with the shredded carpet of wood chips, nor up to the mountains I'd hiked for so many years. But I knew they were there, just like my daughter lying in a bed in a building behind me in a room overlooking a city skyline, a bridge, and the silhouettes of islands far to the south. Dead now.

Had they come into her room yet? Zipped her inside a bag? Or was she lying there alone?

Something shifts. I knew I wouldn't turn back. But I kept walking, just in case.

Finally the back gate. I looked up to the house. There'd been too much dying here. Too many long goodbyes. I squeezed Scruffy between my thighs and pinched the blanket tighter, wedging it inside my zippered fleece. Like a man on the moon, my right arm lifted up and over to release the ice-cold iron latch, pushing it open just far enough. The garden path was longer now. Tiny steps on the concrete. No ants in the cracks. I couldn't recall if I looked left toward the granite rock, "It's All Good," the rock I'd had engraved in Bob's memory. His favourite phrase. Not mine.

Probably not. Today its stark words, black on grey, couldn't be read. Up the stairs, swaying like an elephant, the handrail absorbed my dead weight. Then my hand imprinted, over hers, on the cold brass knob. I turned a half circle to the right. Unlocked.

I walked home. There was nothing else I could do.

CHAPTER 8

No More Walk

Another reason I've come to Mallorca is to walk.

Many do.

The Dry Stone Route runs the length of the Serra de Tramuntana mountain range. It gains popularity with hikers in the temperate fall months. Divided into eight stages, Llucalcari is named in stage five. The path comes out just metres from my front door.

When I'm in the house I hear men's voices, German mostly, amplified in the cul-de-sac.

I only hear them when I'm lying in the hammock, which consumes most of the front room on the top floor. Hammocks, I discover, are difficult to negotiate, this one especially. It's constructed entirely of white sheer netting, with a canopy of white gauze. My feet get lost in the folds, so I always keep one leg dangling out the side, and push against the wall every few minutes to keep something moving.

On good days I rush over to the tiny window, my portal to the outside world. Peer down. The hikers, kitted out in sensible neutrals and sunhats are searching for a path that leads away. With no store or sign of life, they're flummoxed.

"This is it," I call down. I can see them, but they can't see me, which is just as well. "This is the only road." *Then* they find me. They look up and wave in acknowledgment, or lift their hiking pole.

"Thank you," or "Danka," they say.

I join the Saturday Pilates class. Keep the body moving. It's at the coffee social after class when I overhear a woman say, "He died last month of a brain tumour." My ears prick up, as they do now whenever I hear those words, *brain tumour*, unsure if it's pleasure I feel in hearing of someone's misfortune, or the easy temptation to assert my own losses and rob someone from the right to feel pain.

The woman is talking about losing her father. Under my breath, and to myself, I gasp. *How fortunate to have had him for so many years.* But I don't say that. What kind of person would say that?

Bob used to say, "Pain is pain." It's the sort of thing he always said, and why, perhaps, I felt such an attraction for him. His non-judgment. His validation of others' feelings.

But there's a private ranking system nobody talks about that compares the magnitude of our gains and losses: the loss of a child trumps that of a parent, which trumps that of a pet. We're always comparing our griefs. I still do. I have to live in a world without a daughter.

Heartbreak can soften the heart. But I think it's made mine more brittle. The damage, I'm afraid, is permanent.

"Where will you go after Mallorca?" asks my brother-in-law, Graham. He and two friends have flown over from Manchester to run in the annual Palma Marathon.

"South America, perhaps. I'm learning Spanish. To prepare myself."

The day after race day they come to visit me, a forty-five minute drive from Palma. We're all four of us, eating squid-ink paella at an outdoor restaurant, my foot throbbing beneath the tabletop. We've just finished a four-hour hike to Port du Sóller, an ancient cobbled trail built by the Moors. But the main event, it turns out, was the breaking of my toe. An hour earlier at the beach, Graham had accidentally stomped on my bare foot in his hiking boot.

"How about Australia? Do you think you'd go back there?"

"Nah, I don't think so."

Three days on, my foot is a mess. No shoe fits. I can't sleep, can barely get around the house. Stairs are excruciating.

This is exactly what I dread. Confinement. If I felt stranded before, then this was confirmation. I am alone. Completely and utterly alone. This out-of-the-way home had seemed like such a grand idea. But that's me, always jumping into the fray. I was the child who raised her hand in class, whose arm shot up, hard and straight, believing that what I had to say was either essential or correct. Probably both.

Why here? A place so far away from everything and everyone? Not two nights ago a windstorm had knocked out the power. The lights were back on but not Wi-Fi. I just checked. Still down.

Beside my laptop, her jar sits empty.

Ready to fill.

I hobble over to the bed, my foot throbbing. Ask my daughter, "What was it like to know you'd never walk again? To wake up and wonder if this day might be your last?"

In Rachel's final weeks the palliative nurses arranged a day out, at her request. The paramedics bundled her with blankets, strapped her to a gurney. Chest. Hips. Click.

"One. Two. Lift."

The passenger door of Daryl's car was wide open. He held it as they lifted her in.

I climbed into the back.

"Okay, kiddo, where to first?" he said. A stupid question, but she turned to him. Just a bit. Smiled her crooked smile.

Nodding at his suggestions. Looked out the window as he pulled away.

It was socked in and damp; I wish it'd been a nicer day. But you take what you're given. The scenic drive around Stanley Park wasn't very scenic.

A fire truck was waiting outside the house. Daryl pulled up behind. Handsome men. Their short hair, I noticed, was impervious to the gentle drizzle. No gurney, they carried her back to bed. Her smile lingered into the evening.

The next morning was a bright morning. She looked so cheerful. But then this happened.

"Again?"

"No, babe. We can't do that again. It was a special favour."

Her chin dropped. I saw that beseeching look in her eyes, and thought she was going to start crying. Her horizons narrowed once more.

"I'll look into it. Ask the nurses what we can do."

I raised the plastic cup to her lips, directing the straw to her mouth. Applying a dab of Vaseline to a Q-tip, I painted the hard yellow patches on her kissy lips. My heart pulled so tight.

She looked at me intently, her lips moving slightly.

"No more walk?"

She knew the answer but her voice begged for something different. I brushed my bent finger against her cheek, her left cheek. Soft and plump and pink.

"No, babe. No more walk."

I drag out the Suitcase. Open it. Inside is the Ziploc bag that holds her ashes. It's cloudy and pitted and full to bursting. Already, I'm in danger.

Back at the desk, I peel open the seal, *poof*, pour her into the jar, maintaining a steady stream so there'll be no mess. And then I do this. I poke my index finger into her ashes and stir her around.

This.

This is it.

All that's left of my daughter.

I'm standing at the top of the stairs with a bag of frozen peas balanced overtop my right foot. The hate for my whole fucking life echoes back in the hollow corridor.

It's a two-handed job, lifting the icy bag over my head and smashing it to the stone floor. I watch the peas cascading down the steps like a spray of green bullets, pop-pop-popping.

The neighbours hear my scream. The ear-splitting cry. I sense their panic, their deep voices conferring in Spanish, "What shall we do?"

I sit down on the top step and weep. My knees pulled in tight.

Where the hell would I go even if I *could* walk? What am I searching for? Home? Some meaning in all of this? Fuck that.

I look down the marble stairwell, survey the damage. Some of the peas have made it to the hat stand at the foot of the stairs. Their final resting place. Then I'm down the stairs and down on my knees, gathering up the injured peas, apologizing to them for my outburst.

"I lost my daughter," I say, dropping them back inside the severed plastic bag. Call me crazy but I think if I talk to them they'll offer me forgiveness.

Rachel was in Grade 3 when her music teacher recommended she join the Vancouver Bach Children's Chorus. The audition date was June 14, Charlotte's seventh birthday. But we drove the forty-five minutes across town, Rachel and I, so she could try out.

I wanted her talents to be recognized, for her to be singled out. I wanted others to know she'd been selected, to listen in amazement at the news. "She made it."

She refused to sing.

"C'mon Rachel. We've come all this way. You said you wanted to do this. Now's the time."

The lady holding the auditions didn't want to force it.

"It's okay, Rachel," she said. "Perhaps next year."

"No, she wants to do this," I said.

The lady tried again, leaning forward and placing her hands on the keys of the grand piano, then playing the first few chords of "Happy Birthday" to bribe Rachel in. The seeds of sound were moving on her lips.

"Come on, Rachel. Sing." My voice amplified in the church hall. "We're running out of time." (The audition slot was just five minutes.) "When you get back in the car I think you'll regret not singing."

Nothing.

I wanted to protect the opportunity she had to shine. Rachel had perfect pitch. Were she to sing, I was quite sure she would be accepted into the choir. She'd grown up in a house filled with classical music. Beethoven's Fifth. Wagner's *Tristan und Isolde*. And I sang constantly around the house.

"And what will your dad and Grannie say when we get home? They'll say what a waste of time that was, a waste of the lady's time, my time, of how silly it was to have missed such a wonderful opportunity."

I could hardly believe this was my daughter. Growing up I made an attempt at everything. "Becky always has a go," said my mother. So this paralyzing fear, her hesitation, was alien to me. Her back was pushed against my calves, then her face in my armpit.

How could I have missed what was clearly there to be seen? I could have crouched low and hugged her like I always do when she's sad. But my mood was heavy. Heading home, rush hour would be against us.

But I coerced her into singing.

She believed me when I told her I wouldn't leave until she sang. And in that moment I didn't care what the lady thought of me. Or Rachel. And whatever impoverished and ignorant understanding I had of my daughter in those few minutes, I also knew she would forgive me.

She sang. Three lines.

I felt terrible.

We drove home. She said nothing. Which made it worse.

"Say something."

I bring up this story about the audition because I'm intrigued by guilt. My guilt. Now that she's dead.

When she was a newborn, her crying overwhelmed me. When she was only days old, I let her cry too long before lifting her from the crib. She was almost inconsolable. I didn't want her thinking I'd be at her beck and call. Didn't want a spoiled child.

Her father and I were trying to have a little quiet time. He'd rented *Out of Africa*. We were deep into the story. And my bleeding nipples felt like bee stings. Then it hit me. I was a mother. Responsible for her well-being until adulthood. There goes the next eighteen years, I thought. What a burden, motherhood. Even now I'm ashamed to admit my ignorance, my naiveté.

Parenting. We're all scared of getting it wrong. Plenty of days are filled with regret. And heartbreak happens. Disallowing our children their feelings, or changing the subject, wasn't that the usual stuff parents did back then? We can't change what we don't notice.

But a different set of parameters defines the parent of a dead child.

Nothing can be done now. *There's* the grief. You can create memories suitable for framing, but the other kind, the private agonies, I try not to feel anything.

CHAPTER 9

INDECISION

Life in Mallorca is slow. Days stretch beyond the usual twenty-four hours. The question is how best to spend them. How long to sit around doing nothing, at least nothing tangible, without self-judgment or guilt? The beach is out. Everyone's naked. I don't want to be naked. At first I try to make my days feel special. Driving around in the rental car, I explore the northwest coast of Mallorca (a UNESCO World Heritage Site), to accomplish something.

The two-hour hike to Castell D'Alaro offers up a stunning 360-degree view of the Serra de Tramuntana mountains, across the eastern plains toward Palma, and out to sea. The ruined castle perched at the very top was, I thought, a perfect spot to leave some of her ashes, except I had none. I'd left them back at the house. It was my second day in Mallorca. Next time I'd need to be better organized. That evening I zipped the jar, which I'd left on the hall table, inside my handbag. After that I never went anywhere without it.

This wasn't my first time in Spain. My parents brought us here twice on summer holidays when we were young. Packed into the Wolsey, I was wedged between my two older sisters; our father drove the five of us south, through France, over the Pyrenees, then on to the Costa Brava, a place that at the time drew few English tourists. I remember the radio playing Cliff Richard's "Summer Holiday" and us girls singing along, and that for the entire drive my sisters got to lean against a door and look out the window.

For a long-time teacher to live laissez-faire, I was beginning to find out, was agonizingly difficult. There was nothing familiar in the form of my days. Overwhelmed with the enormity of my losses, I head down to the kitchen for wine. Glass in hand, I heave open the front door and stand out on the silent street.

Nothing.

Look at the plant pot by my door. Something is growing, but it's unrecognizable to me.

Summer becomes fall. The November rains arrive. Rarely do I go outside. Knowing such little Spanish leaves me in a more exacting silence. My clothes dry by the fire, draped over the back of the kitchen chairs. Jeans and towels take days. I listen to the winds rising outside. The rain. Water leaks into the art studio. Brown stains smear the whitewashed ceiling and walls. The room smells of damp plaster. I reorganize the thick plastic sheets.

Most nights after dinner, I turn the kitchen chair toward the fire and stare into the flames. I hold the stem of my wine glass between my thumb and forefinger, make tiny rotations on the placemat.

I think about Rachel. How often she and I had sat together at our kitchen table. Commonplace memories. We'd laughed a lot in that easy intimacy of living together. Even, especially, near the end.

It all comes back. The rainy October evening when she, with just one hand — her left — was attempting to chop her Tamoxifen pill in half, to eke out the supply until the next appointment. Her right hand was a lead weight in her lap.

I was over at the counter with a wad of bloody paper towel wrapped around my severed fingertip. Chopping onions too fast. The serrated Cutco knife lay in the steel sink, blood on the razor-sharp edge.

What a fiasco. It launched her into a fit of giggles. Her eyes wrinkled, and she threw back her head. I joined in, the two of us laughing hysterically at the lunacy of our joint afflictions. Rachel bent over now, holding her belly. Jack sniffed at the splinters of a white pill flying off onto the hardwood floor, us both shouting, "Jack! No!"

Relieved by our silliness, he nuzzled beneath his blanket.

On it went. Her flailing with the dinner knife, chuckling.

She didn't question my tears. The cut was reason enough to cry. But I couldn't tell her that the pills, the fourth chemotherapy drug they'd prescribed, were no longer working. It didn't matter if she took one, or a half, or a quarter.

The sight of her trying to save her life, gutting.

Millions of people suffer from depression and I'm one of them. In the past ten years, three episodes. Here in Mallorca I fear another looming. Except this despair is different. The point, best made by Julian Barnes in *Levels of Life*, four years after the death of his wife, is this: "Everything you do, or might achieve thereafter, is thinner, weaker, matters less."

I'd spent so much time thinking about how Bob's death taught me to treasure life, but after losing Rachel, the idea feels unconscionable. Even now I can barely muster the energy to get out of bed.

Indecision. It's keeping me awake. Where to go after Mallorca?

There's a woman back in Canada whose advice I'd come to rely on. At times, depend on. She'd welcome me with open arms, a long, firm hold. Firmer still when I left. From her came a sort of quiet, deep moan, "Hmmmm…," as if she knew exactly what I hungered for.

"I don't know what to do," I say, "or where to go now." I can see her gentle nodding over Skype.

"It happens when you've lost so much. You wrestle with the seductive illusion of certainty."

"Don't we all?" I sigh.

"You especially," she says, leaning closer to the screen.

I list off some possibilities.

"You've got it backwards," she says. "Listen to where your feet want to go, not your head. Get out of your head."

This sounded exactly right.

"But there's another thing."

"Go on."

"I think I know something that others don't."

"Very likely," she says. "Tell me."

"Everyone's waiting for something to be different, for the time to be right. It's a different kind of dying."

She nods.

"That's the problem with breathing," I say. "It makes us blind to our mortality. It's a problem I can't talk about, at least not to strangers."

"Yes," she smiles. "Yes."

There's a knock, hard on the heavy wood of my front door. Embarrassed to still be in my pajamas at midday, I pad down the stairs, crack open the door. It's Nicole, come to pick up her books. The move has done one of us good.

"You okay?" she frowns, places her palm on my forearm.

"Yeah," I lie. "How's it going in Palma? You feeling settled yet?"

"Good," she says, "really good. It's funny, huh? You never know what's going to happen. *That's what makes life worth living.*"

My eyes light up. I remember the sensation: the quick jerk of my neck, my back jolting straight.

"You're right," I say, stepping out of the house.

"Absolutely!" she says. "Who'd want to read a book if they knew right from the start how the story ends?"

She opens the car door, climbs in and starts the engine.

A steady stream of water is cascading onto the hood of her car from a downspout protruding high up on my neighbour's wall. The condensation is fogging up her windows.

"A good story never turns out the way you expect," she says, leaning out the window. "Why should we think life is any different?"

A coastal path connects Llucalcari to the picture postcard bay of Cala Deia. It's late afternoon when I head out. My singular intention is to leave some of her ashes in the Mediterranean Sea. Peering down from the cliff top, I see that the water sparkles, even now in late November. Looking more closely I notice dark patches just off the shingly beach, rock pools below the surface.

Here she is again. She's eleven, sliding off the back of the boat into the deep-sea swells of the Great Barrier Reef, snorkelling ahead of me among giant clams and corals. The swells had made my stomach knot. Wretch.

Rachel went out alone. Three more times.

She didn't need me at all.

Celebrating my remarkable ability to walk, I take a handful of her ashes in with me, squeezing her tightly in my hand and diving down into a subterranean grave; I open my eyes just long enough to bear the salty sting. But as my hand enters the water she's gone, stolen from my grip before I was ready to let go.

What happens now, to her ashes? Will they remain unchanged or do they dissolve like salt in a broth, as if she never existed? Will ocean currents carry her from this body of water to the next?

Might she be here already?

Last year in Italy, her ashes five months old, I'd left her in the Adriatic Sea.

My sister had waited in the car while I ran inside. I left the engine running and returned to our room to grab the cardboard container.

It was my first time doing it. I breathed deeply, like they teach in prenatal class, to steady my racing heart. *Calm yourself. You're not doing anything wrong. Just keeping a promise.*

The beach was empty at this post-siesta hour. Fish soup, *brodetto,* would've been in the making somewhere along this Adriatic coastline.

"Let's go," I said, fastening my seatbelt.

She lifted her sunglasses. "What did you forget?"

Maybe she heard the same hard buzz as me — my heart banging against the doors and windows. I forget what I told her.

"Hey, it's July 1," I said, clearing the air. "It's Canada Day."

Down the windy road, so close to the edge, then under the railway bridge that carries train travellers north from Bari to Bologna.

My flip-flops in one corner of the beach towel, faded stripes of blue and yellow, and Rachel's small daypack in the other, like anchors on the sand. I rubbed my sticky fingers against my damp thighs, coarse with sand and goosebumps. Snatched up my water bottle, poured fresh water into my palm, a tiny pool to wash my hands clean, in preparation. I licked my fingers, then knelt.

I fumbled with the zipper but my fingers were unwilling, as if I'd coerced them into a crime against humanity. Again, I licked them for traction, recoiled, spat the crunchy sand onto the beach.

Inside the tiny front pouch is where I'd stashed them, minutes earlier. A travel-sized portion enough to last me three weeks in Europe. The cardboard shower cap pouch is where I'd hidden her ashes, "Rachel" printed neatly with blue pen in the top right corner. I squeezed the cardboard, midway down, the bird-beak opening wide to reveal a corner of the plastic Ziploc bag wedged tightly inside.

I looked up to check that my sister was still swimming, then dug my hand into the Ziploc hidden inside the cardboard, hidden inside the front pocket. Too well hidden.

The cardboard snapped closed.

An elderly lady arrived. She spread out her towel right next to mine. Smiled.

All this space and she chooses here! I don't remember what she looked like, only that she shouldn't have been there.

I cussed under my breath. *What the hell are you doing here?*

She nodded at me, happy I suppose, to snatch a few minutes down at the beach before dinner. So happy it seemed she might even start talking.

I turned my gaze away. *Lady, you're going to wish you hadn't sat here.*

This is not the way I wanted it to be. But my future hinged on this. A flash of red, my sister's bikini, caught my eye. She was standing in the shallow waves, walking back to the beach. Her body was amazing. Four children had come from it. All still alive.

I yanked on the plastic seal, not caring if the stuff flew everywhere or if I lost loads on the towel. Finally it gave way. I peeled open the bag, just halfway. Reached inside. The gritty dust stuck to my shaking fingers, lodged under my nails, and the wind was picking up, but I couldn't open the damn thing any further and I had to hurry up. I needed so much more, but to expose the bag, to pull it out in full view, was not an option.

"Aahh, that was lovely," Debbie sighed, sitting back on her towel, dabbing her feet dry. She pulled out her book, looked over at me fiddling with something as I climbed to my feet.

"You going in again?"

I bolted down to the water's edge with a clenched fist.

The Adriatic warmth held me. Wading deeper into the luminous turquoise, arms outstretched at shoulder height, one hand scrunched, I must have looked odd. I didn't look back to see if my sister or the old lady were watching. Now I was here. Just me. And her. Yearning for something different.

Should I fling my hand skyward as if throwing a Frisbee? No, too noticeable. Who does that? Do I swish my hands around my thighs as if contemplating the just-right temperature for a swim, then simply open my palms and let her go? Again.

As I spread my fingers, the ashes fell away, dissolving from the creases where they held tight. My words and tears given to the wind. I rubbed my fingertips over my palm. All I held of my daughter washed away at sea.

Just like that.

CHAPTER 10

A Minute Too Long

The death of your child changes everything.

The common wisdom is that resilient grievers are those with the most secure attachments. I had let my relationships atrophy. Friends were active in my life but I was not in theirs.

When you lose a child you live with a uniquely debilitating grief. Her death piggybacked on the death of my fiancé a few years earlier, so I qualified as Master Griever. No surprise that I chose to isolate myself. To be around those whose lives appeared so together, who cheerfully regaled stories of their children's escapades, only seemed to increase my pain. There was a chasm between us. Only a similar grief might bridge that divide.

At work I told no one.

By the fall of 2009, Rachel's tumour was no longer responsive to chemotherapy.

My combined class of Grade 6/7 students had been restorative. Every day we laughed. I didn't want to leave them. Rachel, I felt sure, needed time alone at home. Or at least that's what I assumed, because it's what Bob wanted.

"We'll get an emergency cord," said the community nurse. "Just in case she falls when you're at work."

Not a week later I was called out of my classroom. The next day, the uproar of my sudden dash from school, I knew my hard-fought secret was out.

The teachers had known anyway. I'd stopped singing in the corridors. I dashed from the staff room at lunchtime, my mouth still full. My emotional hiding wasn't new. But I imagined they talked amongst themselves, wondering, *First Bob, then Rachel. How will she hold on, especially through this one?*

Two friends and a counsellor bore the brunt of my grief. I spared them nothing. Deep under the duvet I spoke to Jenny in Nova Scotia. The other was Peter. He was a beacon to me.

After Bob died I never imagined I'd kiss another man, but I'd let Peter do that and a lot more. It was a golden October evening when we'd waved each other off the road at a red light, pulling over our cars into the closest lot. It was still light and the air was crisp. Yellow leaves blew around our feet. We hugged long and hard, a shy, intimate complicity.

"You look amazing," he said.

"Thank you. You too."

Shades held back his fine black hair. The dark eyes, the unshaven, after-five look, the gap between his front teeth, and his smile just as I remembered. Like rain for a dry field.

"So, how's life? How's the guy?" he said. "You married yet?"

I remembered then, it'd be the end of our small talk.

"He died, Peter. Last summer. Bob died."

He pulled open the sides of his creamy leather jacket and pulled me in tight, wrapping me in and pressing my head against his chest. My cheek nestled against the lining, pale blue with tiny flowers edged in black. I breathed in the smell of him, soap and fresh leather.

My desire for Peter never changed. The first man I dated since Daryl and I separated, he embodied a past of happier times. Spontaneity. Fun. Possibilities.

We'd met at a singles wine-tasting event in December 2000. What followed was ten months of intimacy on his terms. It seemed like a small price to pay to be touched.

When he ousted me for the manager of an upscale restaurant, I was heartbroken. But he still called. Often.

"I don't wanna let you go," he said, pulling me in tighter. I let him. I always did. Six years ago, when we'd first dated, it was all I'd wanted to hear.

"This is Jack."

We turned to look at my rescue dog tied up on the back seat, still sitting. The obedience classes were working.

"He's the only man in my life." I wanted him to know.

He slid his hand around my waist. "We should get together sometime. Still at the same number?"

I nodded.

He checked his phone. I was still there in his list of Contacts. But I blushed as I watched his fingers moving, remembering how he used to hold my hand, gently stroking my palm with those fingertips.

So it was here that our connection began anew. For the next two years we dated, in something resembling a "relationship." In all that time he never confessed to love me. And I needed to hear it, believing foolishly that *if he loved me he wouldn't leave me*. Toward the end of Rachel's life, her health so unsettled, the prospect of losing him too teetered on revisiting a deep, dark place. So I stayed. And so, I thought, did he.

After Rachel died, he bailed. I didn't realize. Not for months.

"I'm glad you were with me till the end," I said. The house was empty. My mother and sister had flown back to England just days earlier. Peter and I were lying on my bed. Fully clothed.

"I wasn't," he said.

We never talked about what that really meant. But there's a lot of power in the unspoken. "Will you stay with me through all this?" I never asked, terrified that he might not.

The truth is, neither of us could handle my grief. The more it closed in the further he ran.

"It was always just about you," he told me some months later. He was right. When a person dies, old griefs stir up: other deaths, traumas, shattered dreams. His adored older brother was killed at work eight years earlier by a bullet intended for someone else. But when Rachel was dying I never gave it a thought.

Away from familiar surroundings, I found space for my own grief and was able to open myself to the grief of others. Grief I couldn't see early on but now can.

With a seven-week housesit in Tasmania confirmed for March 2012, and one week until I was to leave for India, I decide to call my friend Anita. My flight to Delhi is booked to and from Melbourne. And Anita calls Melbourne home.

"Wonderful," she says, "I'll pick you up at the airport."

It's dusk by the time we arrive at her home in Port Melbourne. Hers is the centre house in a row of three. A small front terrace is framed by cast-iron filigree, like a trimming of white lace. As we enter, the air is perfumed with the scent of oranges.

"I love to bake," she says, leading me toward the kitchen at the far end of the house. "Mediterranean Orange Cake seemed appropriate."

Like me, Anita sings as she walks. I wonder if I sound so good.

A bottle of red wine sits on the dinner table, open and breathing. Anita supplies me with a key. We practise together in the dark, opening the heavy white wood door.

"The lock can be sticky."

There's an expressive octave in which most people communicate; in some, there's many more. A psychotherapist and a Catholic religious sister, Anita works to nurture the "flame of life" in everyone; her humility is born from a hard walk through fire.

We'd met in Ireland's Shannon Airport, the rain teeming down. She knew, from our time together in Ireland, that my daughter had died. Here, in Melbourne, she tells me about her own grief: in a period of three weeks her nephew, and then her sister, took their own lives. As the evening progresses, I tell her about Bob.

"How did Rachel react to his death?" she asks, her voice so gentle. "Were they close?"

Yes, I thought, they were.

Their shared affliction brought them closer.

Rachel, I can picture, sitting on his hospital bed. The doctor had just removed Bob's head bandage after his surgery. His blonde fuzz was all shaved off.

"Yours is quite different from mine," she said, commenting on his U-shaped scar. She pulled back her hair, traced the staple marks of her own.

"See?"

They smiled.

"Brain tumour buddies."

Bob raised his hand, open toward Rachel. She slapped his palm. Gently.

On the day his staples were removed, the three of us went to the Dutch Pancake House for breakfast.

"This is where Mum brought me both times I had my staples out," she said. "Fifty with the first surgery, fifty-three with the second."

Bob and Rachel sat directly across from each other.

I watched. My daughter and my fiancé enjoyed a camaraderie that defied all logic in a fair and just world.

How, then, to answer Anita's question with the care it required? How did Rachel react to Bob's death?

It's hard to know of course. So I'll speculate.

How does the way we feel about life show up in those closest to us? Rachel had always tried to please me in a way only a child can. Through the loss of love between her father and me, and the strident demands of her younger sister, Rachel remained triumphant in keeping me happy. Not just happy. Sane. But with Bob, I'm not sure. The night they discovered his tumour, she'd hidden down in the basement. I'd heard her sobbing, "It's not fair." I didn't go down to join her. Did she want me to?

Even though she still lived with us at home, working in coffee shops to save money for her travels, I have little recollection of our relationship during the time Bob was dying, or after he died. Not that it matters now.

All I can be certain of is this: for six months she watched him. Watched him swallow temozolomide, the oral chemotherapy drug used for the treatment of an aggressive brain tumour, which she too, in her final year of life, took as prescribed. She watched his physical and then his mental capacities erode. His sporadic confusion, his restlessness, and how, toward the end, he made no sense at all. She listened. She knew what was possible. I think she was petrified she'd lose her mind.

She knew when a brain tumour has stolen everything from you, *almost* everything, and you're offered a chance to make one choice, to take control over just *one* thing, you might take it.

He did.

So did she.

"I think Bob's death made it easier for Rachel," I tell Anita. "I'd like to think it did."

"Medicine."

"Medicine?"

"Yes."

"You want medicine to make you go to sleep?"

"Yes."

"Forever?"

"Yes."

For four days we watch Rachel stir on and off, her body slowly poisoning itself. A torturous wait. Once you've decided, every minute is a minute too long.

"We never quite know the right dosage with these things," says the doctor.

I still don't know how to write about this. About my daughter struggling not to die. Cats and dogs are awarded more dignity. The doctor agreed.

Hadn't she already endured enough? Almost eight years they'd been injecting her. Poking her soft skin to draw blood, inject contrast dye, anesthetize.

Time and again, we're convinced she's fallen into a permanent coma. Then she drags her eyes open. Looks at us. Begins to cry. The medication worked so quickly on Bob. Why not for her?

The delusion that she was in control of her destiny was perhaps the most difficult discovery.

"The swelling will press against her brain stem, choking the neural pathway that makes breathing possible," says the doctor. "No breath, no oxygen, no heartbeat."

You can hardly believe you're willing your daughter to die. But there you are. Doing it.

You have to stay calm. You can't say, "For chrissakes, just get the fucking thing done."

"With Rachel being so young, so healthy, it's…well, her body's fighting to stay alive. Let's try an alternate drug."

It worked. She never opened her eyes again.

On the fourth day, her fingertips turned blue.

CHAPTER 11

THROW AND CATCH

A good many years pass by in slow degrees when nothing of particular note occurs in a person's life. Not even our children's.

It's the reason perhaps that I can't tell you much about her childhood. Until the body blow when everything changed. When she was fifteen. You'd think I'd want to reclaim whatever I could of her early years. Or, rife with vagaries and generalizations, do I consider it all too mundane? Nothing of much interest to others.

To admit that breaks my heart.

Photos help.

She's dancing. Arms high, hips lopsided, lips pursed.

She's three years old, lying back on the sofa with her head on the armrest, headphones on, listening to "The Music of the Night." She'd memorized the lyrics, sing out loud in the car, impersonating the Phantom, leaning into the agony of his pain with an undeniable talent.

She's naked in the cardboard box with her sister, knees tight to the skin of their chests, as if in a boat heading off on a grand adventure. Her age? Why don't I remember?

Australia: a gargantuan snake is dripping down her chest, kind of hugging her waist. She's smiling her flawless smile, composed and calm, holding a length of the reptile like a tray. In another she's stroking a koala, as if it were no big deal. It made me think of how easy she was to love.

If you were to ask her teachers I think they'd tell you that Rachel was "nice," "good-natured," "amenable." That kind of thing. And what parent isn't happy with that?

I could tell you about the way she'd melt when you stroked her back and her neck. "My pussy cat," Grannie would sigh, Rachel's head pillowed on her thighs.

She's sitting beside our neighbour's zucchini, a monolith half her height. Her face. Her keen dark eyes. You'd be blinded from the inside out.

I was.

But then I suppose all mothers must feel that way when they watch their child loving life. Her joy was a kind of glue that kept my husband and me together for years.

Charlotte arrived in our world when Rachel was twenty-one months old. I mention this because much of what I remember in the early years is about mothering two girls. Besieged by work, all I wanted was my daughters to get along. And they did. Any conflict, Rachel gave in. Submission, I understood even back then, was the indispensable ingredient. It made life easier. For me. No arguments to help solve. I could say that I wished she'd been more assertive, but I'm not sure how true that is.

My paradoxical love of, and hate for, bland compliance remains even now.

We have an appalling capacity to see things clearly. As they were. But here, alone and far away, I'm able to really concentrate, to bring those childhood memories back to life, to isolate one from the many. In *The Tao of Travel*, Paul Theroux writes: "Nothing inspires memory like an alien landscape or a foreign culture." I think he's right.

Here's one.

The Emergency admitting nurse, a soft-spoken woman, lifted her glasses to look across at Rachel, three-years old.

"Now how did you get that metal washer stuck on your finger?"

Rachel was eager to tell. She chattered away, wriggling to the front of the padded chair, her legs swaying forward and back, and she beamed at me.

I was in love with her shining life. Imagine. Even here in the hospital.

"Mummy couldn't get it off so we went next door to Maureen's. She tried soap to get it off, but nothing worked." I can see her still — her ponytail, a twisted ringlet flipping this way and that. Any closer and I'd have taken a lashing, the crunchy ends scratching my eye.

My mother used to pop me on her knee, dabbing a knob of butter on my bumps and bruises. But that seems foolish now. An old wive's tale. Still, it was a comfort, and I had no equivalent in my arsenal of nursing children.

"But she gave me this to make me feel better." Rachel showed the nurse a stuffed toy baby lamb, stroking it as she placed it on the table beside the computer.

"So, young lady," the nurse giggled as she leaned across the desk, "when do you expect to receive your first Oscar?"

Rachel sprang back in her chair. Her brown eyes were full and they sparkled. Her mouth was a perfect "O."

You remember those things.

Pixie cute blonde, Charlotte stole the stage. Always it was stories about Charlotte that I heard from family and friends, never stories about Rachel. Our Japanese homestay students played with both my daughters but Charlotte persisted, dragging them into her games of horses and ponies, reading to them, and they to her, for hours and hours.

My father came to visit from England. He would do this trick like he was pulling off his thumb. Rachel, five, and Charlotte, three, watched with glee.

A few years ago I came across a video of his early visit to Vancouver, he and my girls playing throw and catch with Velcro paddles out at Spanish Banks. Rachel lacked the coordination necessary to impress my father.

His booming voice carried on the wind, "Tut, tut. Some mothers 'ave 'em."

But being two years younger, Charlotte's ineptitude was permissible, even adorable. There's Charlotte storming off, with her arms folded tight at her chest and my father is laughing, calling her back. Did he not see Rachel stepping forward?

"Here, Grandpa."

It was around this time when a sadness began to settle in me. The disparity. Affections and attentions shown to Charlotte. Not to Rachel.

In 1998, the girls and I moved to Australia for a year while I was on teaching exchange. Daryl flew out to visit. In Sydney he held Charlotte's hand. She reached out, and he took it. They remained as one for days. It was awful. Rachel at eleven, with her long legs, and her longer legs, no longer qualified for his affections. It was as if she didn't exist.

She said nothing.

Then she lost Piggy in Alice Springs. She didn't lose things as a rule, or have the need for comfort regalia, but Piggy was an exception. A beany made of pink terry towelling had become her new mate. In Australia she took him everywhere. And now he was gone. The minibus had pulled away by the time she realized. She rarely called attention to herself, but that evening, as she threw herself on the bunk, face down, it pierced me.

There are many ways to get attention but only the most obvious wave their arms trying. Rachel didn't.

Some get sick.

Then we notice them.

At four years old, she went to the hospital again.

"Looks like an asthma attack," said the emergency nurse. He hooked her up to a nebulizer, placed the clear plastic mask over her mouth and nose and administered what would be the first intravenous drip of her lifetime.

Three times he tried to find a vein. I left the room.

After the brain tumour, of course, I can tell you everything. Listening now with a special urgency, I predicted her moods, and imagined her thoughts racing and losing. Mostly my heart just ached.

Could we start again?

It was childhood asthma. Triggered each summer by freshly cut grass. The first time, by heaps of fresh hay Daryl had shoved into the homemade bunny hutch. At the end of the year, one of my Grade 4 students had given me a rabbit. It needed a home.

What occurs to me now is this. The stories I'm sharing lean heavily on her ailments, her accidents, her shortcomings. I could go on.

How often is "a lot" when I tell you she came down "a lot" with the flu, with coughs and ear infections? How many falls or accidents are normal? I haven't even told you yet about the scars on her legs. One, on her left, from a horrendous fall on barnacled rock when Grannie had taken her to Cortez Island that summer I was studying at UBC. The other, as she leapt onto her bed, the rigid plastic tail of a toy stegosaurus etched a three-inch groove deep into the soft flesh of her inner right calf. Or about the ten bee stings she accumulated in childhood, seven of which occurred on a field trip to Bowen Island. The boy walking ahead of her on the wooded trail had kicked a nest. She was in the firing line.

What's missing perhaps is my role in all of this. What kind of mother was I for my daughter?

There's no question about it. When our children get hurt or become sick, it's then that we show them an extraordinary outpouring of love and affection, stroking their hair and skin, kissing their head, their cheeks, and their "owies." We snuggle them up, we talk baby-talk, hoping as we do to absorb some of their pain. Isn't it strange to find out this way just how much we love our children? How deeply?

CHAPTER 12

Unforgettable Places to See Before You Die

Two boys emerge from under a bright blue tarpaulin. They've been shouted awake by a man, demanding they start their morning duties. They strip to their baggy white underpants, grab a hose and run a stream of icy water over their brown skin. Shivering, they pull on trousers, their legs still wet. Their sweaters have holes for elbows. They begin to peel potatoes.

It's my first day in Delhi, 6 a.m. and I'm wide awake. So is my roommate. We head out into the deserted streets before the group gathers for breakfast.

"Why India?" asked the doctor back in Perth who authorized my typhoid shot. "Isn't it rather foolish," he frowned, "a single woman travelling alone to such an impoverished country? Have you considered the dangers?"

He wheeled his chair toward the printer, his feet pedalling across the carpet, hand at the ready. "You might contract swine flu on the plane. Only last week, I treated a twenty-nine-year-old man who was raped while on vacation in Bali."

His fear confirmed something I'd noticed in my ten weeks living in Western Australia. Fear was ubiquitous. Not so much fear of skin cancer or shark fatalities, but the dread of a Chinese take-over. Captured on the back windshield of a Perth hatchback, a sticker: Fuck Off: We're Full.

"Oh, I'll be fine," I said, unsettled more by his fears than any of mine. "I'll be travelling with others and don't plan to be out alone after dark."

India? For me it's a longing to gain perspective that I need now, to see hardship and poverty up close and the ever-present veil between life and death.

And the Taj Mahal.

"Take nothing but a camera," says Pravar, our group leader. "Security measures at the Taj are strict, and strictly enforced."

Nailed behind the bus driver is a sign: Prohibited Items at the Taj Mahal. On it: twenty-four pictures (three rows of eight), each circled in a thick rim of red, each cut through with a red diagonal line. Pictures so small you couldn't decipher even one. But I'm sure of this: I won't be the first person smuggling ashes past security.

Pravar had me worried. Dressing that morning, I'd considered stashing the jar in my bra. Or my hat.

We're directed toward the lineups for women: "Indian Women" and "High Value Ticket Holders," then herded toward the latter. I watch one of the female guards shove her hand inside the bag of the woman ahead of me and dig around.

"Your camera," she says. "Remove the case."

Another guard pats down her friend.

My mind is a flurry. How will I explain myself? To have come all this way. I can already see the long rectangle of water that I know so well from photos, and that holds the reflection. I drop my cross-shoulder bag onto the long table, the jar hidden inside an inner zipper pocket, turn away and strike up a conversation with two women in my group.

"Madam, here's your bag."

And there it is, my canvas bag of orange stripes, waiting for me to slip back over my shoulder. Walk on. I bite down on my lip, whisper:

"We made it."

I wish I hadn't gone inside. The smell of sweaty feet is heaviest by the entrance. We walked barefoot on the white marble, a tainted brown. A flowing stream of bodies, touching the walls of a mausoleum built in love's memory. "Move along." "This way." "Keep it moving." Children run around, their voices amplified by stone.

No, the Taj Mahal is much better from a distance. You can see her curves. The garden laid out in four quarters, the pool reflecting her fullness. From far away and from every angle, her beauty astonishes.

Waiting for the right time is problematic. Privacy in famous "places to see before you die" is slim to none. And I'm certain that as sunset approaches, so too will an influx of tourists. I sit on a bench, well back and far to one side, a long bed of deep-red roses just inches from my feet. *This is where I'll leave her.*

To my right, an elderly couple slows down. He points to the bench beside mine. *Please don't sit here.* But she slides her handbag from her shoulder, gathers it to her chest with both hands. He lays his hand on the small of her back. Guides her in.

Now's my chance.

I lean forward.

They sit down.

I lean back.

They look over. We nod. Smile.

David, a member of our group, has a camera permanently slung on his hip. It's the length of his forearm! He must be making gobs of money — a houseboat on the Thames, frequent trips overseas — arrogance in his deep-set eyes and severe goatee. Without consent he makes us a target for petty thieves. Before our two-week tour ends, I'm convinced his fancy camera will have vanished. I'm wrong. He fashions the device with such dexterity; his camera, like a body part, flashes into the open air with a series of running clicks. He captures moments that elude the rest of us.

He sees things we don't.

One fireside evening, lounging around on rough blankets beneath the stars, David and I start talking.

"The pain in your shoulder," he says. "What's that about?"

"No idea."

He'd noticed that too.

It had begun in Mallorca. By the time I arrived in Perth I was barely able to raise my right arm over my head. To undress I'd hang forward at the waist and let gravity do the work. In India, the pain was excruciating, like a shard of glass had lodged in my scapula.

"Ah, it'll pass." I say. "But thanks for asking."

"Hey, I was just checking in," he says. "I figure we all need to nurture, and be nurtured."

"So true." I laugh, amazed by his insight. I'd not pegged him as wise. Or a man of compassion.

Back in my tent, I wondered where I fit myself into that picture. What did "nurture" mean now that she was gone? When home was synonymous with Rachel?

I'd given up so much. Given up hearing Rachel laugh, chatting over dinner, calling her into my bedroom when she came home late. What would I replace it with? There's no mathematical reasoning. No simply loving my other daughter twice as much to even out the equation.

This journey was asking a lot of me. Above all, don't resist what you can't change. There's no comfort there.

Letting Rachel go, a little at a time; I can do that.

Just that.

Some said that Bob's death was like a rehearsal for Rachel's. *You've been through this. You know what it's like.*

In some ways, they were right, I suppose.

Both had a brain tumour in the left frontal lobe. Both lost use of the right side of their body. Her slow decline mirrored his.

But that's where the similarities ended.

Bob had spent his final month in a hospice, a calm space kept cool by the gentle breeze awarded by a corner room. We liked it that way. I spent my days lying in bed beside him. "Feels good," he said, winking. The nurses would smile and shut the door.

A rash rose up on my face, my lips were permanently cracked, I lost weight.

"Have you considered this?" said Carol, the hospice social worker. "That to take good care of Bob you first need to take care of yourself."

I'd looked at her aghast. "Why on earth would I want to do that? He's about to die!"

Bob knew it too.

"Slow down," he said. "Be gentle with yourself. When I'm gone, it's going to be what gets you through."

At the end of Rachel's life, the house was abuzz. Her father moved into the basement. Charlotte returned from university. Nurses and palliative care workers, her friends, her grannie, and my sister popped in and out constantly.

That's when I'd go hiking in the woods. Peter picked me up and off we went. Yoga, too, every week, just as it had been since Bob had died. *Shavasana* and anonymity, the hooks. Often I thought back to Carol's words and knew my leaving Rachel was not a dereliction of duty, but instead, essential for enduring the inevitable blow ahead. I'd read enough literature, too, about the effects of continual stress on the immune system, to know that I was a prime target for disease and accidents.

But no one tells you about the lack of privacy that comes with palliative home care. Doors are always opening and closing.

And because it was Christmas, nurses' faces changed often. I'm thinking of one, a particularly insensitive woman.

"How awful to be losing your daughter," she said, plonking down on my sofa. "I think that must be the worst thing that could ever happen to a parent."

In a house with a dying daughter, I was careful not to shout. My bedroom door made a firm click when I closed it slowly and pushed hard.

Caring for a dying child at home, you're besieged by questions. Hours are unclear. Mornings and evenings indistinguishable. Everyone is talking. It's a campaign of distraction. You must override the compunction to indulge others' curiosity and remember how, to them, your daughter is just a patient who needs treatment.

How's she doing today?

How did she sleep last night?

Has she complained of any pain?

Has anything changed?

What should I give her to eat?

I was thinking of washing her hair today. Would that be okay?

I won't be here for the next few days, but somebody else will be in to cover for me.

One minute you want to scream: "Get out! Everyone get out!" The next day you're saying, "Thank you for coming. I'm so glad you're here."

I wanted more of just her and me. Just as it had been with Bob. Just as it had been for us, since Bob died.

I wanted to sit with her and watch one of her DVDs, perhaps *Zoolander* or *Robin Williams on Broadway*; or look at her travel scrapbooks together; or bake some Peanut Butter Oatmeal Cookies, take the empty bowl into her bedroom, hold it in her lap while she runs her left index finger around the insides, then watch her lick off the raw dough. And later, carry a couple of warm cookies in on a plate, her with a glass of milk and me with a cup of tea, and sit beside her in silence. But none of that happened.

People presuppose that familiarity suggests expertise. It's logical. But the way I see it, getting good at grief isn't like other skills that can be mastered with adequate practice. No. Grief is an experience *out* of time. It's the presence you bring to the dying that changes. I'd found the book *Stay Close and Do Nothing*, written by Merrill Collett, a long-time volunteer at the Zen Hospice Project in San Francisco, remarkably helpful. I first read the book after Bob died, and then again before Rachel. The title is perfect. Listen carefully. Watch. Let them lead you through and you can better intuit who and how to be in the company of the one who's dying.

One night she called me into her room. "MUM!" Her voice a panic.

The commode — a feat of teamwork at nighttime. This one particular night the bowl was missing. I saw it on the floor, but it was too late, and like an accordion folding in on itself, down she went, her rear end slipping slowly through the open cavity. We each looked at the other. And then I saw it, her crooked smile. She'd already forgiven me before I said.

"Sorry."

A hard stream shot to the floor. It splashed against the wood, the trail pooling behind the door. But to see her laugh! Her knees were almost up to her chest now. And me, hopping around on tiptoe to avoid the splashing, screaming "STOP!" scrambling for towels to absorb the flood.

As funny as it was tragic, we hadn't had this much fun in ages. Daryl rushed upstairs.

"What's going on? Is everything okay in there?" I could barely catch my breath over his frantic knocking.

I didn't want him to come in. I just wanted him to go away. It was just the two of us feeling silly. Almost like life used to be.

"Fine. We're fine."

It's believed that a dip in the Ganges liberates one from *Samsāra*, releases one from the endless cycle of death into rebirth.

Varanasi, considered the most sacred place on earth for Hindus, is listed in Rachel's book. Fires there burn twenty-four hours a day. Unlike North America, where death is hidden, grieved solely as a loss, here in India it's considered a shedding of a worn-out body: a time to celebrate.

I'd seen pictures of families carrying loved ones down to the river on funeral pyres, a bamboo stretcher, their bodies covered in orange cloth. On the ghats, men performing the rights of the dead: bathing, drying and cremating. Fire purifying the body. The spirit freed as the skull explodes from the intense heat. Men shovelling burning embers into the Ganges. A Hindu ritual dating back five thousand years.

Women are absent. It's believed they bring too much sorrow to the proceedings. I get it. In Vancouver, I couldn't go to Compassionate Friends, a grief support group for those who'd lost a child.

Rachel had been dead for eighteen days. Everyone had gone. My sister Debbie had flown back to England, and three days later, my mother. They'd planned it that way. To leave me gently.

The house was silent. The whoosh of the furnace the only sound. At the kitchen table I sat slumped over a placemat and looked down at Jack stretched out asleep. How had all this commotion been for him? A rescue dog with cinnamon freckles and floppy ears of crushed velvet, in the early months I'd considered returning him to the shelter, and eventually that's what I do.

My focus shifted to the vase of flowers outside on the deck. Red gerberas mostly, a bouquet from the parents at my school. Gerberas were Rachel's favourite flower, and red her favourite colour. Whoever designed the bouquet had stuck a diamond sequin in the stamen of each bloom. That's where my focus landed — the sparkly bits.

And then I realized that for so many years I'd been thinking: this can't be my life, this accumulation of loss. I picture it now: the deck crowded with people at Bob's small celebration, just eight months after we'd bought the house. And now here we were, some three and a half years later. Just me.

A knock at the front door.

"I know I shouldn't do this," Daryl charged in, "but I'm not sure what clothes she should wear..."

"Stop!"

But it was too late. I already heard what he was about to say.

More harrowing still was the image of her body in a morgue. A drawer opening. A sharp tug. An ice-cold wall of drawers. Her name on a label. My daughter. There with other dead bodies in a hospital basement. A ghostly white. Rubbery. People touching her dead body. *Where did your life go?*

I got up, started to wash the dishes, chewing on the soft flesh of my inner cheek.

We'd already decided Daryl would be the executor. Only the executor can pick up the ashes.

"You'll need to sign off on all the paperwork," I said. "Close her bank account, file for a death certificate, return her Care Card and her driver's licence."

"So, I'm sorry to ask again," he said, "but what do you think she should wear?"

My hands stopped moving. Everything stopped. Blood froze. But the tap kept running.

"Look in the black garbage bags," I said, not able to turn to face him. "Debbie and I sorted her clothes. In the laundry room."

He took quick steps, like a gallop, going down.

"I'm keeping her passport," I called out to him. "And her tap shoes."

Ten minutes later Daryl was at the head of the stairs.

"I've taken what I bought her for Christmas," he said. "The Roots sweatpants and this T-shirt." He opened it up, held it by the shoulders to show me.

"What do you think?"

The slanted hemline, the silvery design, wasn't her at all. I figured she'd have never worn it anyway. I didn't want these to be the last clothes she'd wear, but I wasn't going to argue.

In Rishikesh, further upstream, I am sitting on a grey, sandy beach. Beside the river a shirtless man sits cross-legged, meditating. To my left, two hippie-types, mid-twenties, laugh and share a smoke. To my right, a young child runs between her parents, who are splayed out on an overturned rowboat.

No one would notice me enter the holy water, or care what I was about to do.

The deed done, I squat on the beach and talk to her. Tell her where we are. Bone white particles settle on the wet sand. Some cling to the surface like pollen, illuminated by the dirty sunlight. They look so dead just lying there. A panic wells up. What part of her body am I looking at?

How I wish I'd had her courage, the courage to surrender my aversion to pain. I wish I'd pulled my pants higher and taken her deeper into the waters where the river flows. But I'm afraid of the deeper currents and of what the water might do to my skin. I'd gone in barely mid-calf.

Maybe it'll take a decade or her lifetime again, twenty-three years, for her ashes to reach the ocean, be reunited with the souls of centuries. Whom, I wonder, do we swim with when we take a dip?

Caught in a reverie, I'm jolted awake. Something is pressing against the base of my spine. I keep my eyes firmly ahead, imagining who, or what is behind me now, and how I'll escape.

A black dog, a homeless stray resting his chin on his outstretched paws, looks up as I turn. His snout is like Mac's, our old border collie. The scruff of his neck, thick and oily. I slowly massage his matted coat as he closes his eyes, lowering his head back down to sleep.

CHAPTER 13

STUCK

High into the barren Himalayas, Bhoupi looks back at me through the rearview mirror.

"I can't find the gears," he says, slowing to a crawl, "only third." It's not the worst news in recent years but we're precariously close to the edge and I can feel my belly knotting up. Bhoupi is my driver for the week. My third and final week in India.

"Tell me," says Bhoupi, "why do you want to go all the way to Shimla?"

"A picture of the Viceregal Lodge," I reply.

He says nothing.

"My father was a captain in the British Army. He told me that officers went to Shimla to escape the summer heat in Calcutta."

"It's a long way for just two days."

"Well, I thought I'd check it out."

Still nothing.

I don't have the heart to tell him the truth. With seven days to kill before my next house-sit in Australia, Shimla was a random choice of destination.

Safety was never a consideration. The driver. The route. The car. The folly of taking advice from a man who knew a man who drove me in his tuk-tuk to a back alley travel agency that first morning in Delhi.

So where does this come from? This devil-may-care attitude? This aversion to being careful? Couldn't I have stayed in Vancouver, grieved my losses in familiar surroundings like so many others choose to, or have to? No, that would've been squandering a life, not saving it. The truth is I've grown more reckless, understood perhaps only by those who've been up close to the death of a child.

The mountainous pass turns out to be more construction site than road. (Cement manufacturing is big business in this part of India.) Orange dust obliterates what I'd hoped would have been magnificent views of Himalayan valleys. Entire mountainsides are covered with neatly spaced terraces. I see them only through a dusty haze.

"What are they growing?"

Bhoupi shrugs. "Potatoes. Some fruit."

The higher we drive, the worse the road. Bhoupi swerves to avoid the deep ruts molded in the dirt, like gullies.

That's when the gears go.

Bhoupi makes a phone call, hangs up, but says nothing to me. I don't trust him. A short, pudgy man with shifty eyes who yesterday concocted a tale about road tolls and taxes imposed by each of the provinces we drove through, all illegitimate.

"See the world," my father said. "It's the best education you can get."

He'd tell us tales of far-flung places he'd been stationed during his time in the army, his voice charged up. By the age of nine or ten, I felt sure that a passion for travel was a guarantee of my father's love. It's what I got from him, but possibly more.

He'd beaten the odds. At sixty he was diagnosed with an acoustic neuroma, a neat, plum-like brain tumour with well-defined borders, the good kind. Eight hours of surgery and it was gone. To look at him you might think he'd suffered a minor stroke; the slightly lopsided smile.

Neuroscientists claim 5 percent of primary brain tumours have known hereditary factors. It's not a topic I've ever raised with my father. Why would I? If mutations from his genes were encoded into my daughter's DNA, plaited into her cells even before she was born, what would it matter now?

Bhoupi spots a man working under the hood of a car. He pulls off to the side. I pull out my book about goddesses.

Across the road, men, twenty or so, sit around white plastic tables drinking beer. I feel them staring. A schoolgirl and her father walk past the car. He tugs at her arm, recoiling like I'm a plague. It's jarring. All I want is to get back to Delhi, my ticket out. Trucks barrel through, swirling up clouds of fine powder. None stop. Why would they? Bhoupi's right. I should've stayed closer to home.

So why exactly *am* I here? Alone. In India? Following my heart? Indulging my siren-call for adventure? Hardly. Or am I enamoured by the idea that someone, when I tell this tale, will be impressed by my courage? It's easy to do, mistake recklessness for courage. Or might this entire expedition be nothing more than a grand display of theatrics acted out on a global scale. Yes, it's all of the above.

In the family hierarchy of five, I was on the lowest rung. My survival was based on being noticed. There was the long blonde hair but it wasn't enough. More often, I was noticed for my physical incapacities, and frequently reminded of how much slower I was to master the physical skills my two older sisters had apparently acquired easily. Unable to catch, throw or hit a ball with any semblance of accuracy or consistency, I was among the last to be picked for team sports. At home I was a crybaby and a sore loser, hopeless at swallowing pills and keeping secrets.

It's here, sitting in the back seat of a broken-down car, where for the first time in all my time away I feel, not brave, but rather, irresponsible and foolish. "Only you," my mother would say, "could get herself into these situations."

My mother loved my stories. I told them well, dramatizing for added effect, and she'd always laugh. I loved it when she laughed. I knew she'd pass the story on to her friends, faking exasperation at her youngest daughter's antics.

She didn't laugh much when I was a child, even though I tried to break the tension.

Sunday dinners, my father played a game with us called General Knowledge. It would start at the dinner table.

We sat in our assigned places, unfolded our white seersucker serviettes, the interlocking stripes of peach and lime, tucking them firmly inside the necks of our matching Sunday school dresses. Our mother had used her new Singer to make them. Always desperate to be the first of his three daughters to answer, I wriggled with excitement and sometimes my napkin fell to the floor.

My father prepared himself a shandy, a mix of beer and lemonade, and took his place at the head of the table. With the fresh English Leather soapy smell of his clean, still-damp hands, he unpacked the knife and steel from their black leather case. The lush purple folds inside gave them a royal look, as if only special people could use them. I watched in adoration at his swift strokes, the steely edge needed to carve the leathery roast.

The windows fogged up as my mother lifted the lid from the steaming dish of vegetables. I thought the green and white Denby was boring and ugly. When I got married I'd choose something much prettier.

"Shall we begin, John?"

The air was charged. "Elbows off the table, girls."

Some Sundays, as my mother carried the dishes in from the kitchen, there was a slight delay before she could join us, as she was still stirring the gravy, wanting it to arrive at the table steaming from the boat. Our father grabbed his cutlery in fisted hands and banged the ends onto the table, his impish chanting,

"Why-are-we-waiting? Why-are-we-waiting?" My sisters and I joined in.

And on it went.

I could never be sure if at any moment my mother might break. Her lips pursed, her nostrils opening like wings, she'd exhale sharply. Sometimes she stormed out of the room. None of us knew what to do.

But I'm a good girl. So I would placate. My chair was closest to hers.

"A funny thing happened in church today," I'd say, or "Do you want to hear the new song we learned in Music?"

Sometimes it worked. I always tried. Always.

"I was worried the car wasn't fixable," I say, leaning forward as Bhoupi fastens his seatbelt. "I was scared we might be stuck here."

He smiles at me in the rear-view mirror.

"This is India," he says. "Everything is possible."

It must be a sign.

In India, everything is a sign.

Two things happen in Shimla that I'll never forget.

First, the Viceregal Lodge is closed. ("It's Holi Festival," said the ticket agent.)

Second is mailing a gift to Charlotte.

A green-eyed girl with long blonde hair and a knock-out smile, Charlotte is a head–turner. Always has been.

She was twenty-three when I left. I've stopped calling her my younger daughter. Now, Charlotte is simply "my daughter." Her photo, slipped down the outside pouch of my handbag, is slightly wrinkled now. On her hand, Rachel's Celtic ring, one of the last things that carried her sister's touch. "I never take it off," she told me. Sometimes I think Rachel's memory binds them more tightly than if she were alive.

In the months after Rachel died, I'd been to visit Charlotte often. A university student living with her long-time boyfriend, she'd filled their apartment with pictures of her sister. One, with Rachel's arms flung forward over Charlotte's shoulders, caught my breath. The outpouring of affection wasn't Rachel's style, but in this photo her eyes are ablaze. It made me feel she wasn't quite dead.

"I don't know how you do it, seeing your sister's face all the time." (There were no pictures of Rachel in my apartment in Horseshoe Bay.) In this, it was her courage, not mine that was called out.

But how do you reconcile losing a sister so young? You don't. It showed up in IBS and a flare-up of chronic anxiety.

Two months after Rachel had graduated from Grade 12, her team of doctors scheduled her for six weeks of radiation treatment, I changed jobs, and Charlotte, at sixteen, a tempestuous straight-A student, went to live on a horse ranch four hundred kilometres from Vancouver.

She never came home again. Not to stay.

I never asked Charlotte how she felt about my leaving Vancouver to go travelling overseas. Why would I? I'd have gone anyway. She understood that her mother had lived through a decade of agonizing stress. "And stress can kill you," she'd said.

No one said it. It was just implied. "Aren't you abandoning her?"

No, I'd tell them. All I was abandoning were the years of being afraid.

Still, I wonder how to live here on this side of the world but still show my love there, in Canada.

I'd phoned Charlotte from Mallorca.

"Does your dad phone much?"

"Yep, every week. Sometimes twice."

A relief. It's what I'd asked of him.

And on another call: "Hey, get this! You're older than your sister ever was."

"Thanks for that, Mum. Great way to start my day."

Tactless, I know. A result of too much free time: tallying up Rachel's days on the planet — 8533. It sounds like a lot.

"How about you fly here for Christmas? My treat." She'd turned me down. I bought her a puppy instead.

And in Rishikesh, the funky yoga pants and baggy shirt I felt certain she'd love, were the reason for my visit to the tailor. India Post requires packages to be stitched in cloth.

I sit across from the tailor, his first customer on this freezing cold morning.

He flips through remnants of white cotton, searching for the right-sized piece. Between us, only the sound of his scissors, cutting cloth.

As he slides the fabric under the foot of the needle, his feet begin rocking the treadle, forward and back. The ragged-edged fan belt. His Adler machine, a dinosaur.

It starts to snow.

He slips the clothes into the smaller bag, then the larger. Snug, like his scarlet turban. With needle and thread he stitches the final seam, passes the package across the table, hands me a pen. A red pen.

I print Charlotte's name and address in big block letters. C-H-A-R-L-O-T-T-E. My heart aches to make her name. The letters bend into the padded cotton. Some, I go over a second time. And I want nothing so much as to curl up and be stitched inside, flown back to Canada to see her again.

The tailor lights a match, takes the flame to a thick four-sided red crayon. The red drops melt onto the cotton. He pushes a wooden stamp into the pool of molten wax, sealing it for India Post.

The bell dings as I close the door behind me.

A swoosh of conditioned air welcomes me to Delhi's Indira Gandhi International Airport. The automatic doors slide open to a shiny, sterile world of neutrals, glass and generic space. I like airports. They're full of people who don't belong.

I splurge on a private, soundproofed, windowless room. A beautiful lady in a dark uniform and a shiny bun unlocks the door with a special card. I wheel my luggage down the carpeted hallway, trailing behind her.

"Wake me in four hours."

I pull off my filthy sandals, drape my papery Levi's over the suitcase, and release the crunchy sheets from their moorings. Inside, my knees pulled in tight, I retreat deep under the covers from the madness on the streets of India. The dead cow on the outskirts of Pushkar, its entire head cavity empty. The roaming dogs had each taken their turn.

Cocooned in a teensy black room in an airport of a vast country, a ball of body, a bump in the bed.

Take a pin, stick it in a gigantic canvas of the world, and there I am. I pan out onto a global image of land and water, of millions of people who call this planet home.

There's a long, deep sigh, a blissful stillness, as if a child's birthday party is finally over and everyone has gone home.

CHAPTER 14

THE SUITCASE

Without a home, living light is a necessity.

For twenty-six months my home is a suitcase. All said, it's packed and unpacked around 250 times.

And let me tell you, living out of a suitcase can be a real pain. It's not for everyone.

Empty, the World's Lightest Expander IT-0-2 suitcase weighs only 2.7 kilograms (meaning the contents could never exceed 20.3 kilograms).

Here's how I prepare for moving day.

On the day before my departure I slip clothes off hangers, empty drawers and throw everything on the bed.

"Here we go again."

It's not that I mind really. Sometimes I'm happy to be leaving.

I make piles, folding each item neatly to fit into one of the five Pack-It Cubes.

Some days I roll. Others I fold. Sometimes I hear myself talking to my clothes as I pop them in, zip them up. "There you go," like I'm tucking them in safely for a long drive home. Often it's easier (but not easy) to chuck out a T-shirt or two, if the armpits are smelly, or if I don't wear it enough. When you live out of a suitcase, you redefine "essential."

Sometimes even 23 kilograms weighs too much. Surely the less one has, the less one has to fear losing. But still I pack the contents of my changing self to my maximum weight allowance. Why is that?

Here's why. We hold on to our stuff like we do our stories. Stories need cleaning out too. We forget that. They become us. If we let them.

And we let them.

One Pack-It Cube is for exercise gear. It's the most difficult to zip up. Eventually the mesh tears, and like a weeping wound, stuff starts oozing out.

There's the black nylon drawstring bag for dirty laundry and a small zip-up bag for electrical stuff. Another for jewelry.

An assemblage of stuff. Just stuff.

One bag holds a Ziploc containing Rachel's ashes.

About now I have to stand up, stretch my legs, make a cup of tea, go to the loo, look out the window, start vacuuming, anything really to break the monotony.

I never really count how many times I do this. Or how long it takes to pack up. But I'm always careful to leave the home with no trace of my ever having been there.

Perhaps it's true that movement only has meaning if you ultimately have a home to go back to. I say that because always, at the end of every stay, I feel agitated and gloomy. Over time I recognize the tears as a response to saying goodbye.

I lock the door, drop the keys through the mail slot and off I go, dragging my life across driveways thick with gravel.

"Bye house."

CHAPTER 15

ONE CAT

When you look on a map for the city of Launceston, you see it in the north of Tasmania, the island shaped, some say, like a woman's pubic area. The island state lies to the south of the Australian mainland, separated by Bass Strait. A ten-hour ferry ride from Melbourne or a one-hour Virgin flight will get you there.

Devon Hills is close by. All homes have acreage. Most mornings a wallaby is dead on the road.

Can a home be a home in just minutes? I decide it can. For eight weeks I call this home.

I smile all the time here. A silly grin.

It's the wind rustling the gum leaves, the wallabies bouncing through. It's standing on the rocky mound as I hang my laundry, the warm wind coming from every direction, tossing my hair, spinning the clothes dry in minutes. It's miles of unblemished beauty that the floor-to-ceiling windows offer up. It makes my throat tickle.

I look upward and outward. At last, the alchemy of absence begins to heal something deep in my bones. On the fridge, I hang John O'Donohue's poem, "For the Traveller."

> ...you will discover
> More of your hidden life,
> And the urgencies
> That deserve to claim you.

Caring for others' pets has run the gamut. But one cat, Moonbah, changed my life.

It's March in Tasmania, early fall. Warm days and cool nights, cooler still in the remoteness of this hilltop home.

There's scratching at my bedroom door.

"Moonbah, cut it out." But he doesn't. He's a cat. I grope for the bathrobe hanging on the hook of the door, pull on the thick striped tiger socks and turn the knob. The blackness hits me first. Then the icy cold. Through one slit eye I catch Moonbah's profile leading me to the back door, then I negotiate the passageway back to my bedroom, grumbling.

That's when I see the sky.

Before sunrise it's a full canvas of purple, bright with stars and the Southern Cross. As the sun breaks over the edge of the planet, bands of black and vermillion splash southward from the east; a quadrant of stripes burning up the skies. At dawn, a heavy fog tracks the river, carving a path through the valley and drowning the fields in white oblivion. A soundless landscape broken by a rooster's "cock-a-doodle-doo." I slide open the heavy glass door and step outside, place my hand over my heart to calm its wild beating.

There's a bedroom upstairs but I don't sleep there. Some mornings I climb the wooden slatted stairs. They creak like those in my old house. The timber-framed roof rises like a church steeple and although it barely seems possible, I step out onto the deck to bask in a view double the size. Giant skies, which restore a measure of silence to my world.

My wish is to stay here. Stay, and never grow tired.

Moonbah is my wake-up call.

In *A Grief Observed*, C.S. Lewis writes, "In grief nothing 'stays put.'" A welcome paradox.

For so many years I've strained into spring, tentatively awaiting the worst. This March (fall in Australia) something new takes seed.

I'm overcome with joy.

A joy I haven't known in years, not since all the losses began. Joy!

I want to shout it from the rooftops.

A shocking but guilty revelation out here on the other side of the world, in a house not mine.

Joy is possible in the world of grief. Claim it.

A joy that makes me weep and laugh and stand and sit and dance and sing to the cat, bursting through my days over and over.

Sometimes it takes a great sky to find it.

"I realize now that everything's a choice," said a friend whose wife had been dead a year. "Absolutely everything." He's right. I know it. Rachel, choosing at the end when and where to die, helped me choose how to live. Taking nothing so ordinary as walking or talking for granted.

My life now.

My life then.

Is this joy, me loving again? Learning it back into my bones had at one time seemed impossible. But something shifted. I begin to mourn my losses in a new way. A *firm persuasion*, Blake would call it. That living with joy is the best legacy of love.

Is it because I've done what I set out to do? Followed my heart? Kept her travelling? Has leaving her ashes helped restore my faith in the world? Has a renewed sense of being in control of just this *one* thing allowed me to turn a corner? And this. Was this joy mine alone? Or was it Rachel's too?

Grief is so complicated. Paradoxically, it's only because of Rachel and Bob that I am here. This debt of guilt tempers my joy. Not a day passes without holding these two opposing feelings.

Joy.

This home invites it in. Most days I let it find me. Others, I'm upended. A thump to the side of the head, as if I've just heard she's been killed in a plane crash.

No, joy, now that she's gone, might always be just a hair's breadth from what it once was. How could it not? Reduction is the language a grieving mother learns against her will.

Most things change, but I don't think this will.

Her first sky burial comes at Cradle Mountain National Park. Jacquie has flown out from Perth, so we go together.

The wind is fierce. Greedy.

"Stand clear, Jacquie."

My eyes are watering. I barely have the lid off before she's gone.

Jacquie shouts after her. Something like, "Keep going, Rachel."

We huddle behind a rock and pull out the lunch we've packed. I'm grateful that she is with me. Even so, the sandwich is hard to swallow.

There are so many things we get to love. So many things that get to love us. With Moonbah curled up in my lap, my love is for this quieter, calmer version of the woman who eight months ago had left it all behind.

The fig tree in the inner garden is heavy with fruit. Every morning I pluck a fig and carry the warm weight, heavy and suggestive, in my palm, walking now without effort. I leave it on the sassafras countertop. It smells sweeter, warm. A backdrop of autumn grasses seems to sashay in the wind, as if to music.

Isabel Allende's *Aphrodite* sits on a side table. She lost a daughter too. The book rests on my lap as I read the view. One I commit to memory.

There's no need to move from my chair. It's all there, the shivering river, the long tendril-like fingers of shadow creeping over fields, singling out goats and sheep and cattle.

But I slide open the heavy glass doors and step barefoot onto the warm paving stones, tiptoeing across the prickly grass, and throw her into the fountain grasses sloping to the valley below. An entire jar.

"All this is yours now."

The prosciutto crackles beneath the broiler, filling the room with a meaty burn. I pull the wrapped figs from the oven. Thick slabs of home-grown tomato, overlapping rounds on a white plate, and cracked pepper from a mill.

The rooster crows, and outside, a robin models his tangerine chest to the woman in the window. I feast on my life.

CHAPTER 16

TRACK 2

Some people say I'm living the dream. On a perma-vacation. Some are curious. Some inspired. Some, judgmental, say something to the effect of, "Must be nice to just take off like that."

My unconventional lifestyle suits a few yet seems to hold great appeal for many, men especially; any who long for the exhilaration of life on the edge, closer to childhood freedom.

"You're so strong." Strong! The word comes as a surprise. For so long, weakness had been my wrecking ball. All the self-recriminations, the days and weeks absent from work, the heartbreaking knowledge of brain tumours and dying that had no application in the outside world.

I'm not one of those who rallied to find a cure for brain cancer, nor did I become an activist for doctor-assisted suicide (but I should have). Nor did I seize the opportunity with those thirteen-year-old students in my classroom, to bring them into a deeper appreciation for life and death, and dying, that teachable moment ignored because the teacher was unsure of whom she was trying to protect.

I want to tell people it's a kind of loose strength. A way of stepping forward, about doing what you think will help ease the grief, about not knowing and then doing something anyway.

Some live vicariously through me. I get it. Adventure and novelty often trump the bedrock reality of the daily grind, seducing us into feeling more alive.

They see in me perhaps the willingness at least to pull it off. The common course of life, no longer mine. But it makes me laugh.

For so many years no one would've wanted my life, my marvellous misfortune.

Others are puzzled. "I don't know how you summoned the courage to leave in the first place. I could never do what you're doing." Or, "Don't you want something more certain, more permanent?"

They're the ones who thrive on daily rituals: opening the same front door, seeing familiar faces, TV shows, their pets, just as I once had. All rituals of reassurance.

The same ones who've clearly stated their wishes in a will: burial or cremation. Who've named where they'd like their body laid to rest. The plot of land, the headstone, their favourite font; or the others, who name the special place they'd like their ashes to be scattered. I'm in that group too. Except now none of it matters, only that I tell Charlotte, "Do what you want with my ashes. Whatever will bring you peace."

In a world that prefers easy explanations, I become unexplainable. Living in transit, an act of resistance. Isn't it what we all do when we run out of options?

People ask my friends, my sisters, my mother.

"Where's Becky these days? Still house-sitting?"

Most are completely unaware of the transience one must accept in moving every few weeks from house to house. It's exhausting. I had no influence, no real sense of belonging. Nobody remembered my name. Occupying the blind spot in people's lives, I was conspicuous only because I was unfamiliar.

Without an address you lack a reference point on which to organize your life. Try creating a mind map — HOME — on an imaginary sheet of A4. Not the shapes on paper (though I try that too — the size of each circle relative to the length and frequency I'd slept at any one place). It isn't possible. Not without an image of where I'll return to, or when.

Simone Weil says, "To be rooted is perhaps the most important and least recognized need of the human soul."

Home, I come to realize, needs to be viewed differently. It doesn't have to be a singular, identifiable place. People shape themselves to the homes they make. The nomadic have survived for thousands of years.

Our homes in transit: Rachel's in a jar. Mine in the suitcase, seeking new homes for us both. Each time I find a new home for her, I find one for myself in the timeless border connecting us.

The gravitational pull is believing you're in the right home at the right time.

This is her rightful inheritance and my obligation. It requires profound devotion.

This journey isn't a vacation. Quite the opposite.

Grief changes the narrative of your life. It helps to clarify a vision about the commitments we want to make.

I wanted none.

I'd known for a long time. Even before leaving Vancouver. *Quit teaching.*

"What do you do?" It's a common question in early conversations. Teacher is the quick answer, an identity easily named and known. And one I loved. A lot.

In 1976 there were three alternatives proposed by the careers teacher at my grammar school: nurse, secretary and teacher.

Acting was my real passion, a Julie Andrews wannabe. At high school I'm the girl who entertains: on stage, on the bus, at home, admired by my full command of an audience. The skill was there and I knew it. I'd won my high school drama prize but failed to get into London's Royal Central School of Speech and Drama.

"The results don't matter," said my mother. "All that matters is that you had a go." Her love for me was never contingent on my success. But I imagine she breathed a sigh of relief. It's hard to make a living as an actress. But she never said so. Not to me.

So like my mother I chose a career in teaching.

I was eighteen. I thought I knew so much.

When I immigrated to Canada in 1982, a newlywed, the only teaching jobs in BC were those in remote communities.

For six years I worked in the investment business in downtown Vancouver, first as a desk trader and then as an administrative assistant for a group of wealthy stockbrokers.

In 1989 the BC economy, and the birth rate, turned around. They were desperate for teachers, and I returned to the classroom. A year of being a stay-at-home mum was not for me. Plus the house renovations had gone well over budget; we needed the money.

Teaching fed me in surprising ways. At thirty-one and a mother of two, I was without question a better teacher.

But all these years later, I can't be sure when exactly my well-crafted teaching life took a detour. When, precisely, I became burned out at work in others' eyes. Felt more like a liability than an asset.

In Tasmania, away from the classroom for almost a year, my focus softens. My gait slows. A calling to live life on my terms, not a life regulated by school bells, is what matters now. Let others cling to the seductive powers of control. I'm done with that.

Yet, if not teaching, then what?

Narawntapu National Park on Tasmania's north coast is a strange, alien landscape, as if the only constant has been, and always will be, change. Her ashes like asteroids pit the bleached sand. Mini-craters. Then she's gone, swallowed up between ripples. The wind grabs the rest.

I notice a broken post in the sand dunes. TRACK 2 is seared into each "wing" of the metal sign.

Is it a precursor? An endorsement, for some other future?
TRACK 2.
I decide yes, it is.

My resignation letter made reference to the brevity of life. The letter, I am told, will be read aloud to faculty: teachers, teachers' aides, and administrators, clerical staff, past and present retirees, at the end-of-year retirement function.

"Life is fragile. For some, shockingly brief. Sadly, and far too often, things have to fall apart for us to know this. I was forty-eight when my fiancé, Bob, died. We'd been engaged for eight months. Everything I was so sure would happen, didn't. When I was fifty-one, my daughter died and my world shattered.

Death shook me. Brought it closer.

What if you died next year? In five years? Ten? What do you want those years to look like?"

For those contemplating retirement, I hoped my letter might loosen the hold of "just one more year," the pull of a plusher pension.

I want to tell them about the phrase imprinted on Tasmanian licence plates: *Explore the Possibilities.* About how I'd taken a permanent marker and written in huge letters on a kitchen cupboard of Bob's and my home: "Forever is composed of nows." Words by Emily Dickinson, which shaped our final days together.

Bob used to say, "Life's an illusion." It's only now I understand. Life always has other plans for us. We surrender an old self to something larger.

Or we don't.

CHAPTER 17

FINAL BOARDING CALL

Here's some one-line truths:

- She slathered popcorn with melted butter and brown sugar, caramelized in the microwave.
- She was easy to please. Eager to please.
- She loved the long days of summer, of hanging out at the beach with her friends. (But then who doesn't?)
- She had "moves." And a wicked memory.
- She didn't drink (prohibited with seizure medication). Travel was her wonder drug.
- She was born when I was twenty-eight. I breastfed her for one week.
- She liked the badges at Brownies, the prescribed activities.
- Her eyes were laughing eyes. Wrinkling at the edges, they'd roll shut as her head melted backward.
- I made it my secret mission to make her laugh.
- Monday nights we'd head down to the basement to watch *24*. Every season.
- Contact sports weren't her thing. She played soccer in Grade 1. The coach rarely called her on to the field.
- She was no great fan of mornings; I would often leave her to walk to school. (Charlotte was always ready at the front door.)
- She loved a long, cold glass of milk.
- She could appreciate jokes at her own expense.
- She was four months old when I returned to work.

- She hated commotion.
- She spent hours watching late-night TV: Conan, Colbert, SNL. Jon Stewart was her favourite.
- She said "Yes" to any offer: the orchestra with her grannie, or a walk with the dog and me.
- In her Grade 8 yearbook, she was voted "Most likely to be a model for Roots."
- She loved flying.

I'm at the Melbourne Airport.

England is my destination. Ahead of me are twenty-seven hours of suspended aviation, with only one layover in the United Arab Emirates. Inside a white plastic "Recycle Your Phone" envelope, I've sealed up Rachel's mobile phone. On it, her voice: "Hi, this is Rachel. Please leave a message." I head across the street, my heart pounding, and drop the envelope into the mailbox.

Starburst chews are my flying candy. A pile of waxy wrappers will be scrunched at the bottom of my handbag by the time we take off. But it's when I pay the cashier in the airport lounge that I see it. The jar. The jar in my handbag is half full of ashes. This has never happened before. I've always been so careful to make sure it's empty when I board a plane.

Border security in Australia is hard on illicit activity. I'm aware of that. Not once in these nine months of travelling have I checked on the legality of carrying ashes.

I can see myself being pulled off into a small room. Questioned. Detained.

"If you want to carry cremated ashes on this plane, you need to have the appropriate paperwork," they'll say. "And this jar. Has it been authorized as a suitable container?"

What will I say?

"Well, no. In fact I have no death certificate, no letter from the crematorium. I've never checked my air carrier's rules and expectations, as advised. Nor declared her cremated ashes on any form."

I could say I didn't know. But that's lying.

It's why I didn't brandish it around, my telling people what I was doing until after I'd done it.

"Isn't that illegal? Leaving her ashes everywhere?"

"Too late now," I'd say.

This is where I am. This is what I do. Her ashes: her dowry to the non-human world.

Suggesting that it's a sustainable burial practice is a moot point.

No, human ashes, I think it's safe to say, freak people out. Watch their reactions to talk of dying. Notice their aversion to the word "death." It's too close a reminder of our own mortality. Hollywood touches on the topic only in comedies.

I was above the law, apparently. But that's the thing with grief, mine at least; you don't seem to care too much about what's right or wrong. A young adult, Rachel had hardly got started. There'd been no booze, no cigarettes, no addictions that I knew of other than an unbridled passion for *Lord of the Rings* and for travel.

I'm still sitting by the check-in desk on the upper level, my eyes glued to the Departures screen, wondering what to do with her ashes before I go through security.

EY0461 to Abu Dhabi starts flashing: Go to Gate.

Not to bore you with the details, I go the cigarette route. Step out into the dark night onto a concrete deck, eye level with the neon sign *Welcome Back to Melbourne,* and pretend I'm putting out a smoke. It feels terrible leaving her like that. Listening to the bones crunch beneath my hiking boot.

Dying at twenty-three was the worst thing *she'd* ever done.

My mother is celebrating her eightieth birthday. Debbie, my older sister, has arranged a family gathering in the Cotswolds.

In the days leading up, the pace has been fierce. Someone stirs the soup. Someone lays the table. Someone complains about the lack of hot water. Someone opens the wine, leaves the bottles to breathe along the length of the harvest table. Someone checks the time and channel for the next episode of *Downton Abbey* that the twelve of us will watch later.

"You can't just keep travelling, expecting others to let you stay with them." My sister ties on an apron, checks on the potatoes. "Don't you need to get a job?"

I look at her with spectacular admiration, wondering if she can ever give herself a rest from managing. But where would I have been had she not taken over in those early weeks after Rachel died?

It's a fair question. By anyone's standards, ten months is a long time to live without an address or a "proper job." Perhaps she assumed it was a lifestyle that'd claimed my heart. Why wouldn't she? I was always happy on the road.

"Don't think I haven't thought the exact same thing," I say.

Everyone wants to know how I am. Is she still the same outgoing girl we knew? Or a mother bereft? It started years ago, this silent surveying, wanting to see the changes Canada had made on me and where my loyalties lay.

For twenty-four years I called England home. Land of Hope and Glory, country gardens, Yorkshire pudding and gravy, Marmite, Monty Python and The Beatles, roundabouts and the quintessential cuppa were the scaffolding of my formative years.

Saturday afternoon, everyone spills out of the rental cottage to wander the lanes of Bourton-on-the Water, a picturesque village in England's "green and pleasant" land. Some head directly to the local pub; others just end up there. I hold back until the house is empty and make a break out the back door.

All the planning and togetherness, and I bail. This family gathering to celebrate the birthday of a mother, a sister and a grandmother is the same weekend Rachel would have celebrated her own birthday. Her twenty-fifth.

Did she remember her last birthday? The gift she opened? A pair of grey cotton sweats from American Eagle.

To Rachel, Love Mum xxx.

If you were to see the pictures of her sitting on our back deck, wearing the dollar store tiara, blowing out the white waxy candles — a two and a three — you'd never have suspected anything but total faith in her team of doctors to keep her alive.

I had fretted: what do you buy your daughter when you know it's her last birthday? How do you watch her rip it open, knowing it's you who'll be wearing them for years after?

I'd tried them on, just to be sure.

Around the time cocktails would be served, guilt carries me back to the cottage.

"Where've you been all this time?" my mother asks. "We didn't see you anywhere."

Suddenly I'm overcome with sadness. Not for me, but for her. I'd given no thought to how my travels might be for my mother. A woman derailed so easily by bumps in the road, she'd had to endure this transient lifestyle I'd chosen to ease my pain. Nor did I know her grief when I left England back in 1982, a new bride. Or her grief now, at losing her first-born granddaughter. How must it feel, at eighty, to have outlived your grandchild?

"Cheers!" says Graham, my brother-in-law. "A toast to Eileen. To absent friends."

Everyone raises a glass, stares down the table to where I'm sitting. I'd been unusually quiet throughout dinner. Had anyone else noticed I'd stop talking before I finished a sentence?

Days later, back in my mother's Leicestershire home, we tour her back garden like we always do, squatting beside the fish pond, searching for tadpoles beneath the lily pads just as my daughters had done, at six and seven, when we'd come to visit my family in England.

My mother cups her palms around a pot of heather, the veins on the back of her hands well-defined now beneath her translucent skin.

"*Erica* in Latin," she says. "Rachel's middle name."

I remember now, how I'd sprinkled some of Rachel's ashes into that pot when I'd visited England five months after Rachel died. Unsure of my mother's reaction, I only told her as we were waiting at the airport for my flight back to Canada.

She smiles down at the pot. "I talk to her every day."

CHAPTER 18

MILES TO GO

It's little wonder I travel. In transit you belong nowhere. Suspended mid-air, in line at the border or bobbing around at sea, you're unclaimed, neither here nor there. Time is suspended.

It's the same with grief. The world distorted and warped, it's easy to lose your bearings.

Often the conversation goes something like this:

"Where do you live?"

"Canada."

"Nice."

"But your accent. Where do you come from?"

"England, originally."

"Okay. I'd guessed Australia."

"But right now...I don't live anywhere."

"Aah."

They nod, mildly confused.

Yet, in a stateless state, there's no holding back.

On good days I smile a lot. Ask questions. Sing out loud. You may think me a tad too conscientious.

On bad days, or in the company of a person who suggests you're "doing the *Eat, Pray, Love* thing," or someone who dispenses a litany of complaints (petty, you think) about their partner or the food served on the plane, you let them have it. The whole tragic story. The one, despite my best efforts, I still hold on to, because like a battle scar, it sets me apart.

The urge is strong to correct their notion of your good fortune, or their bad luck. Unsuspecting strangers who sit beside you (big mistake) must yield to the bizarre truth of the double brain tumours.

"I was a lucky child though."

You look so harmless.

Such deceit in a smile. But then death is a treacherous subject. On really wicked days you throw in:

"Imagine? Ten days after we'd moved into our first home. That's when they found his tumour. One day we were looking for an architect, and the next, a neurosurgeon. And a grand mal seizure, just like my daughter."

On occasion, you turn the knife.

"We'd only be engaged for two months!"

You marvel at how masterfully you can silence a stranger, their tear-filled eyes proof of your success.

"He only lived for six months after his diagnosis." A tilt of the head, a shrug of the shoulders, then you go back to your book. Gloat.

But no, you still weren't done, your elbow now nudging their arm.

"Sometimes he'd say, 'Hey, Rach, we're brain tumour buddies.' They'd reach across the kitchen table, 'High Five.' But I didn't think it was very funny."

How do these unknown reserves of bad energy take seed? When does bitterness become your particular currency of grief?

Over time I realize that my intention is to throw them off on a bizarre trajectory, just as I had been. I told them so that they might go home and ferociously love their life, their family, their job, because that woman on the plane, or ferry or in the café, really shot from the hip about grief. Could have really complained but she didn't. She seemed to love her life.

"Your home is your journey, and your journey is your home."

It's May 2012. Two days after landing in Vancouver, I take my car out of storage and drive to Charlotte's house in the Kootenays, listening to a CD by Jim Hollis.

The drive from Vancouver on Highway 3 is almost eight hours depending on how often you stop. It's nothing short of spectacular. The sun illuminates everything: the trickling roadside falls, the raging canyon waters. I keep my windows rolled down.

I stop close to Osoyoos, yank the wheel toward a patch of loose gravel, a quick-and-dirty lookout. Step out of the car. When I lift the lid from the jar, it's as if Rachel's life rises up like an all-powerful genie, and I'm hit by a wave of unspeakable sadness. My throat, a vise. The tug of it.

This is my daughter.

That's how it happens. One day it's a privilege; the next, abhorrent.

I leave her beside the lake where we'd camped a few years earlier. I notice the weight of my legs as I climb back into the car. The heavy *thunk* of my door. My heart, a slug. I pull away slowly. I always pull away slowly.

"Did you have a good drive?" Charlotte asks, welcoming me into her new home, offering me a cold beer.

"Yup, lovely," I say. "I left some of Rachel's ashes beside Osoyoos Lake, where we went camping with Bob. Remember?"

She walked away.

But I kept on.

"A duck swam over to welcome her back."

Charlotte, like many others, assumed that once my jaunt overseas was over, my heart would be restored. I'd find an apartment, a job, pull my possessions from storage and claim my place in the world. Rooted at one address. Then she could say, "This is where my mum lives."

That was my original plan too.

But that was almost a year ago.

I didn't want to stop. Charlotte found it unsettling, worried that I might have lost myself in the saga of Rachel's ashes.

After returning to Canada I continued to house-sit. For the next fifteen months I drove around in my little Honda Fit, with a basket of spices on the back seat, never quite knowing where I'd find the next house-sit or whom I'd next visit. Worse still, I kept waxing on about how much I enjoyed it.

"You're so different now," she says. We are sitting on her deck, waiting for the burgers to cook through. I've been back in Canada for one week.

"Dad thinks so too."

Your dad? What's he got to do with this?

It didn't come across as a compliment but rather, pejorative; that she and Daryl were a team now and I was on the outs.

My life at this juncture was disorienting. I got that. I had been a responsible, working mother, who shopped, and cooked, and paid her bills on time, but now I was a drifter, hard to pin down.

My departure, as I saw it, had been an epic display of courage: the extreme lengths a mother must go to survive the worst heartbreak. I wanted to teach my daughter this one thing I'd learned from my travels. To reconfigure life is what I'd set out to do. And I still had miles to go.

Apparently, since my departure, she and Daryl had become closer. A lot closer. Resolute, he'd become her constant. He'd phoned and visited often. Our Skype calls, though hours long, were rare.

Had I made a fatal mistake? Was that mother part of me I could least afford to lose, lost? Had those words of Ram Dass played out against me in my absence? "When someone we love dies, we get so busy mourning what died that we ignore what didn't."

I had no way to describe the remodelling of my life. No language she would understand. How could she? Even I was unsure. All I understood of it was this: finding ground again after losing so much takes time. Time to remember what we loved, and how we loved. Who I was is no longer who I am. How do you explain that?

Homelessness was my life. And I was in love with my life.

CHAPTER 19

COME TO NEW YORK

How often do we ask someone if they have children? More often than you can imagine, when one of them is dead. I can give you this piece of advice: if you ever decide to ask this question, prepare yourself for any response.

Sometimes I want people to know my daughter has died. I want their sympathy, and to watch their response. Their reactions: mute sadness, fingertips covering the mouth, lips slightly parted, then the sharp inhale of breath, the wet eyes. "I'm so sorry." Sometimes their entire face changes. It's hard to describe the look, but I am privy to that look by virtue of "my news."

"When did she die?" some asked. I could've said, "Just after the earthquake in Haiti," but the countless deaths didn't register much on my radar. The one child you make is so much bigger than the two hundred thousand you didn't.

Nobody messes with a grieving mother.

The man in the neon yellow vest was tucking a parking ticket beneath my windshield wiper as I dashed out of the Greek bakery.

"Don't! Please." He kept writing. "My daughter's brain tumour is back." And just like that, his hand froze.

"This baklava's for her," I croaked. "Please."

He let me off. So did the bank teller. She could have called security, the way I screamed and swore about the "stupid, fucking rules."

It's not really forgiveness. Not really. I am a woman wielding an assault weapon.

It's strange, but my feelings about sharing "the news" I still find confounding. Who wants to be the bearer of a grim tale? My voice will get shaky when I tell about it. Equally possible, I savour an evil delight in inflicting pain, a mere fraction, after all, of what it was like for me, her mother.

Mostly it's just sad. Their day ruined, or mellowed perhaps, by the loss of some other mother's child. So often a jealousy stirs in me that I can't fully articulate. Something perhaps like their child would be spared because mine was not.

After Rachel's first brain surgery, gifts arrived: dinners, stuffed toys, movie tickets, a breakfast basket left on the doorstep.

With Bob's brain surgery, a second wave of generosity. An all-expenses paid vacation at a resort on Vancouver Island. Dinner at the restaurant where, three months earlier, we'd got engaged.

"They need to help," Bob said. "They don't know what else to do."

Dinners again in Rachel's final weeks, left on our front doorstep below the note: "Don't Ring the Doorbell." After Rachel died, a week-long retreat in Ireland — seeds of a new life — gifted by some very generous friends.

Some might think how lucky I am. Some, how unlucky. No matter, that's not really what I want to talk about. What I want to talk about is the charity. I didn't want it. Once, fine. But not a second time. Not three times. Couldn't someone else be the unfortunate recipient?

Yet what really surprised me was how much more charitable people were than I'd ever been, or thought I could be. Had these events not been so catastrophic, I'd never have made this discovery. And another thing: how tragic that we only come to know the extent of others' kindness through disaster.

"Come to New York," said Meg. "Anytime."

In the fall of 2012, between house-sits, I accept her offer.

Meg had been the last one to join us in Cottage Seven. The day's events were already underway when she pulled open the door on that rainy Irish morning. Thirty of us, elbow to elbow, journals on laps, were listening to David Whyte as he read his opening poem. I turned to see the brazen soul who'd shown up late on the first day of our week-long retreat.

"Sorry," she giggled. "Stuff, you know."

Her long auburn hair was still wet. You could see the combed lines against her scalp. Her glasses were steamed up. Even then she was laughing.

For six weeks I live with Meg in her Upper East Side apartment. She loves my cooking, and me. Every evening she uncorks a bottle of red in appreciation. I write. She plays Debussy, Mozart and Chopin on her grand piano. There are random conversations about what God might be. Most nights we read aloud a chapter of *The Tao of Pooh*, one of us sprawled out on her stained leather sofa, the other on the inflatable bed. Mostly we laugh. Always there's a hug, "Good night."

We talk about the things that have changed us.

"I was on the forty-seventh floor. I watched the second plane go in."

She gazes into space. The sky of grey confetti. Battery Park. Watching the first tower sway, then right itself. The blackout after implosion. Her eyes glaze over, locking in on a corner of the ceiling behind me, both of us spellbound. The days after, photos plastered on storefront windows, "Have You Seen?" The silent inventory of folk stepping into the elevator. Check. Check. Check.

The double brain tumours. When shall I tell her?

Operating on the assumption that people can only handle so much bad news, I never mention Bob. Not after Rachel died.

My fear is that you might run away, assume that you too might be cast with a similar affliction, just by association. Only when I feel confident in the future of our friendship do I disclose the whole truth. It's deplorable, my logic. It's like he didn't even exist. A man I loved, sidelined, so that I might salvage some hope in any future friendship.

A daughter dead at twenty-three, and a fiancé at forty-eight.

Lives half-lived.

Gone.

It's a crippling reminder of all that I've lost and can lose again by allowing another in. My heart won't endure another loss, another *having to go on*, having to make it a part of me.

No one knows I feel this way. Most think I have my shit together, that I'm "living the dream." I earned that high school drama prize for good reason.

Rachel loved New York. I imagine where she might have walked, what she might have seen: The harpist by Bethesda Fountain, beside her upturned hat, "The World Needs More Bach"? The violinist, an elegant woman with silvery hair pulled neatly into a French knot? Donate fifteen dollars and get a CD. The saxophonist beneath the bridge, mindful of the best acoustics?

She'd come back to Vancouver with a silver "I ♥ New York" bauble from Bloomingdale's. For years it was the first decoration she hung on our tree. I head to Bloomingdale's to buy another. Why? Was I entertaining the possibility of one day celebrating Christmas again?

Walking home, I pass a vendor cart where a Japanese bride in a poufy white dress, a gabardine coat draped over her shoulders, is squeezing ketchup along the length of a bun. And suddenly I see it, that picture in our photo album: Rachel holding a hot dog up to her lips, the cheeky smile, anticipating the first bite. I can't help but wonder if I'm standing in a place where she once stood.

Travel, like grief, asks how much we can surrender to the unknown. Always it asks, *what do you want to let go?* I'm thinking of a tree in Central Park. Behind the Dodger blue sky, its trunk and branches appear black. I sit beneath it. Unscrew the lid. It feels like taking a pinch of rock salt between my thumb and forefinger, then sprinkling her into the pot of some global stew.

Days earlier the New York Marathon had been cancelled because of Hurricane Sandy. Barricades had been erected but runners showed up regardless. Nobody had taken the fences down. Behind me, runners kept running. Why was I surprised? The people of New York are notoriously resilient.

Strolling in Central Park on my last day, I see a French couple waving and pointing at a piece of paper, trying to make sense of their map.

They call me over. "Excusez-moi, Madame. Fifth Avenue? Le Guggenheim? You know?"

"Yes, I know." I smile. "Come with me; I will show you the way."

I lead them out, past the contorted chain-link fence of a baseball park crippled by ninty-mile-per-hour winds.

I forget exactly when I tell Meg about Bob. Only that she hugs me, then thanks me. How often, I think, have any of us been thanked for our grief?

I know this: for survivors, death is a long affair. Our grief continues indefinitely, and what dies is our belief that we cannot bear the unbearable.

I donate my boots — Rachel's black Ecco boots — to a woman who lost everything in Hurricane Sandy. But my motivation is selfish, too. It keeps Rachel walking the streets of a city she loved. And like most New Yorkers, I understand that every new beginning starts with a retail experience in footwear, so I buy a new pair of boots from Harry's on Broadway. They have buckles running down the outer edge and a small heel. They fit better.

CHAPTER 20

UNFORGETTABLE PLACES TO BE AFTER YOU DIE

Virgin America 744: San Francisco to Seattle, December 2013.

As always, I'm the last to board. One of the last. I like it that way, as if flying were no big deal.

"I think that's my seat, next to yours," I say.

In a flash, the man, a spitting image of Johnny Depp, is standing in the aisle beside me. I can hardly believe my good fortune.

"Here," he says, "let me help you with your bag."

"Oh, it's okay. But thanks anyway."

We settle in together. We search for my seatbelt wedged between our seats. My fingers almost touch his jeans.

I try to read my book.

"So where do you live?" he asks.

A tickle in my throat, I can hardly wait to give him my answer. Surely he'll marvel at my transient lifestyle.

"Well, nowhere permanent right now. I've been house-sitting all over the world for the past year or so. I've just finished house-sitting for friends in Berkeley for the past month."

"That's the best way to live," he says, slowly brushing his goatee with thumb and index finger. "Home is wherever you are, and whoever you're with."

He holds my gaze. I marvel at all of him: his hair pulled back loosely in a ponytail, his fine-knit, pale-pink sweater. His silver earring. He smells so good. He has to know he's a doppel-ganger of the Hollywood actor, and I wonder how much of who he is has been created to perfect the illusion.

I could've told him why I was homeless, but he didn't ask. No one ever asks. But then, did I even want him to know about my daughter? Her ashes? Her homes? My homes? The reason for my self-imposed exile? And what would I have said even if he did ask? Grief renders you homeless? That you launch yourself into a new life or die in the one you have? Or at least, that's what I needed to do. Might he think it morbid? Or on the contrary, be impressed by my courage?

Things were going so well between us, I thought it best to just say nothing.

I mention this story because at the start of my travels I made a commitment to never check-in online. At the airport I take whichever seat the airline assigns, trusting it's where I'm meant to be. It's a novel concept and quite thrilling. Another first step in surrendering control. Often it means taking the dreaded centre seat between the window and aisle. Alone, on uneven terrain, chance encounters are far more likely. I love it: the possibility of meeting not one, but two strangers. Stumbling into and through little moments of realization, "alone" resonates with everyone.

"When I'm with you," he leans closer, his words filling up the narrow space between us, his mouth almost against my cheek, "you're at home."

I respond with a fit of schoolgirl giggles to hide my sudden flush.

What, I wonder, will happen when the ashes run out? Will I stop travelling? Will my grief have settled? Found the proverbial closure?

"Maybe it's time to leave them all in one place," suggests my friend Jenny. "Get back in the classroom. Schools need teachers like you."

I understand her concern. Might all this be an unhealthy attachment blocking my way forward? Clearly, I'm not ready to contemplate such a single defining act. How will I keep her close when there's nothing tangible? I wrestle with these questions.

At one time I consider travelling to all the places named in her book, *Unforgettable Places to See Before You Die*. A silly idea, I know, as if by starring every page in her book, then what? She might pop back and pay me a visit, and we'd celebrate together that we'd accomplished some imagined duo feat?

No, Bucket Lists are nonsense. A checklist we can tick off that masquerades itself as the necessary prerequisite to a well-lived life is surely a ruse. In this greedy world it's easy to believe that too much of life is just out of reach, elusive, only for the world travellers: a measure of wealth. But we've bought into it. Sacrificing time now for time later.

Here's the truth. So much beauty is stitched into what looks "ordinary" from the outside. In searching for beautiful places to leave Rachel's ashes, my focus had changed. Now my eyes locked in on the splendor of shape and colour, of form and light; at one time all quite unremarkable. And another realization: when Rachel no longer exists, I catch myself thinking, "I have to like this for her." Rather like an expectant mother eating for two, my attention is amplified and magnified. It's the grounding in extreme gratitude.

So why on Earth would I want to confine her to the parameters dictated by a book? No, ours was a different tale. One created by a mother, for a daughter. I'd call it *Unforgettable Places to Be After You Die*. Places exclusive to the two of us. Places where I felt her spirit inhabit mine. But I'm kidding myself. She was young. She'd have gone to the places tourists go. Not where I've carried her.

Sand is the perfect vanishing act. Carmel, the chosen spot. Beside me is a white cardboard box. Inside is a slice of pumpkin cheesecake warming in the sun.

"Hey babe," I whisper. "We're at Carmel."

"I have dessert," I say, reaching for the box. "But I know you can't eat it…things as they are."

Twelve years ago, in the summer of 2000, during the long days of our month-long road trip in the Western US, my girls and I were growing tired. Eager to push on to San Francisco before dark, we'd missed Carmel entirely.

We camped instead at Big Sur, a fierce wind blowing in straight off the ocean. Deafening. I'd opened the trunk, was pulling out the tent. Rachel and Charlotte were grabbing at the bag, pulling on the drawstring. They knew the routine. Ground tarp first, then pegs, then tent, then more pegs. It was maybe the twentieth time we'd pitched this tent.

The ground tarp, a green hexagon of cheap plastic, was useless. It flapped and folded in the cracking wind. Its corner peg holes had ripped and torn away. Nothing we tried could secure it.

Hammer in hand, I yelled out to Rachel, "LIE ON IT."

"WHAT?" She turned to Charlotte, then back to me. Shrugged. I tried again.

"LIE. ON. IT."

She must have heard, because she raised both arms above her head in a giant V. Off she went, diving into the centre, spread-eagled. Her five-foot-nine, thirteen-year-old body splayed out, as the tarp snapped around her long, skinny legs, wrapping her up like a parcel. She was laughing wildly. We all were.

I unlatch the hooked S-slot of the cardboard box, wipe the white plastic fork against my rolled-up jeans. Take a bite. Swallow. Barely. I lick the fork. Close the box. Prepare myself.

The beach is empty, at least where I'm sitting, but just to be sure I look around anyway. I always do. I hear the cracking sound of wind and kite, a young man tugging at the blue-ribboned cord of an airborne stingray. I can see his face. There was, I thought, nowhere else in the world he'd rather be.

Unzipping my bag, I pull out my little jar and empty all of it onto the sand.

Running her through my fingers, as if through her hair, as close to me now as she was as a child on my lap. You could count to ten or infinity and never find her.

Virgin America 755: Seattle to San Francisco, March 2013.

A Hindu monk has the window seat. Decked out in orange robes, his head is clean-shaven, a string of dark wooden beads around his neck. I notice his fidgety hands on the latch as we touch down on the tarmac, waiting for the "ding" to authorize release of the seatbelt.

Then he's up, his tall frame contorting beneath the overhead bins, leaning over like I wasn't there, and craning his head down the centre aisle, "Why does this take so long?" His accent was Eastern European. Bulgarian, I think he said.

I close my eyes. His robe brushes my face and his knee digs into my thigh, and I really should say something. But he's struggling. His metal-rimmed glasses have slid down to the tip of his nose, and on his temples are beads of sweat. His accent, like grief, emphasizes all the wrong moments.

"This is taking so long."

We're in Row 25, buddy. This is how it goes!

Arrogant, perhaps, to think the impatient monk can learn a thing or two from me, about how so much of life runs contrary to what we plan or expect. But this woman sitting beside him is, ironically, the one supremely at peace with the here and now. A deeper version of the woman who'd left her life behind almost eighteen months ago, a woman who could "handle things" after all. A woman who had traversed a great distance, and in Rilke's words, could "move in such submission through the world."

Death is the natural order of things. None of us know how long we'll walk on this planet. But who wants a life based on death to understand how it guides their future? Not me. But it's what I've got. It makes me feel proud, and mildly virtuous.

But I've seen that wisdom can come from unexpected sources. Here's what I've discovered: my negative first impressions of people keep proving wrong. On the contrary, they are oddly instructive. Take Bhoupi in India, who I quickly surmised as dishonest, and Nicole in Mallorca, who I'd thought, initially, to be standoffish. David, too, I'd judged imperious. It takes months of travelling to notice that they reveal something in me.

Charlotte once told me, "Rachel worries more about you than she does about herself." Perhaps. And Rachel's comment to my friend Cathy, just two months earlier: "Make sure my mum has a good time at the Winter Olympics."

Could it be that Rachel thought me unable to "handle things?" Or was it that she chose to die unburdened by worry? Hers? Mine?

The butterfly of hydromorphone in her upper arm she self-regulated to relieve her pain. She rarely pushed the button. At least, that's what she told me. Was it recognition of defeat or another kind of insane courage?

When Jim, the palliative care social worker, introduced his student-in-training, she reached out her arm to me to extend her sympathies.

"Get away from me," I snapped, hitting away her hand. What did she know about losing a child?

I spun around. Stormed away.

Picture a four-year-old, her face painted like a cat. She's striding down a grassy slope, then climbing onto the outdoor stage at the Salt Spring Island Summer Festival. Reaching up for the microphone.

"I want to sing," Rachel says, interrupting the man mid-sentence. "I want to sing 'Twinkle, Twinkle, Little Star.'"

Daryl and I were flabbergasted. A week earlier, during Parents' Day at her dance school, she'd hidden under my chair.

She's ten years old, making dinner. As she dices a jalapeno pepper, the juice shoots into her eye. Moments later I arrive home, see her head over the sink. She's splashing cold water from the tap into her burning eye. Is this what happens when you insist on your children helping out with tasks at home before they're ready?

As adults we had this "thing" we did, she and I, when the movie credits rolled. I'd pick out foreign names, or names with puzzling letter combinations, and sound them out, rolling them off with bravado. She'd laugh. It was a game we played. Expected over time.

I could tell you about her annoying teenage habits, how she smeared strands of her long, dark hair on the tiled wall of the shower, or how she scraped out the dirt beneath her fingernails as we sat at the dinner table, flicking it onto the hardwood floor, but how does that help either of us?

Why do I want to recall these events with such pinpoint accuracy?

What would her life have looked like without this?

Without the brain tumour?

Without me?

CHAPTER 21

Rachel's Ashes

Winter 2013, my house-sitting roster looks like this:

One month in Duncan on Vancouver Island.

Eighteen days in Edmonds, Washington.

A week at my friends' home on Whidbey Island.

March, in the Kootenay town of Nelson.

A circuitous route that approximates an anchor of sorts; all are towns in the Pacific Northwest where I think I might one day choose to settle down.

Beside Kootenay Lake, sixty-five miles long, I lay her out on a rock stack built precariously close to the edge. Rocks snapped clean like brittle toffee.

I feel the wind whipping through, and shift. Suddenly a memory: the book *Millicent and the Wind,* by Robert Munsch, a bedtime favourite. And I welcome this; it lights me up. It's the story of a young girl who, in her mountaintop home, befriends the wind as her playmate.

Then it comes to me. The wind wants to find her. Find Rachel. It's asking to be heard, to be remembered.

Don't stay here on the rocks.

What's clear to me now is this: perhaps it was me, and not her, that wanted not to be found. I wanted nothing to touch me.

I think I'm coming closer now to finding her.

I looked for beautiful places to leave Rachel's ashes, and I found them. Some days I'd gone hunting, a kind of goal for the day. More often a place just stopped me.

But you don't think you'll grind ashes into a log stump, like you're filling an open wound with wood putty and a screwdriver. You don't think you'll dash into the middle of a traffic circle on a busy Saturday afternoon and toss them into a dried-up fountain overtop a puddle of stagnant water, moldy coins, a crushed paper cup from Starbucks. Nor do you imagine you'll shove them into a mound of cedar wood chips, warm and damp and smelly like vinegar. "I'll put them in here," I thought.

Yet in the winter of 2013, that's exactly what I did. It's what drew me in: decay and disintegration. Not beautiful, or conducive to my goal to "keep her travelling," but places blurring the line between living and dying, between shape and shapelessness. Not that I noticed at the time.

I threw her over the Kinsol Trestle, because I love bridges. The perfect engineering of line and angle, it's one of the highest timber railway trestles in the world. I watched her go over, bending first as if in a dance, then plummeting as powder does, in no particular rush — and so like Rachel in her old body. Tottering through slushy ice to the other side of the bridge, I looked down, as if in a game of Poohsticks, I might see a trace of her floating downstream.

In the centre of Edmonds, the Gazebo is a local landmark where four roads conjoin at a traffic circle. In England we'd call it a small roundabout.

Weekend shoppers who flocked here for a perfect Pacific Northwest getaway, or to attend one of the free seminars at the Rick Steves' Europe Travel Centre, may have seen two women, sisters, perched on the Gazebo's sharp-angled base, the one in the plaid coat fumbling for something in a shoulder bag she couldn't quite open. No one would have seen what we saw as we leaned over the edge. They wouldn't have heard the low moan over the sound of traffic.

Osborne Bay Park, that's where I jammed her into the log. There was nothing delicate about it. Her tender beauty, camouflaged in ash, was already gone.

But I remember it because it took me so long to leave her that way. It was so cold outside. I wanted to tuck her in tight so she wouldn't come loose. Logs had been washed in on the high tides of the Strait of Georgia. Most were stripped of bark. Burned, not by fire like my daughter, or by uncertainty, like me for so many years, but by the earth's other destroyers: the salted water, the UV rays, the hard-hitting wind. One orange cedar exposed its cutting edge skyward. That's where I left her.

Nothing can fix what is foundationally irreparable, but rituals help.

If I've learned nothing else about grief, I've learned this: It didn't matter whether I believed leaving her ashes around the globe would recalibrate or restore some equilibrium to the skewed axis of my world, only that I made it a ritual. The repetition makes it work.

My powerlessness to change what could never be changed was, at last, redemptive.

It's strange how familiar the jar of ashes had become. Tucked inside my handbag alongside my wallet, passport, my lip chap.

At one time I'd wanted nothing to do with it.

We are all bodies in the world. Her body took me travelling. At last, I realize this is a possession of mine, and that, in so many ways, she has been lost to me again and again. The shape of her true anatomy. This is what this whole journey has been about. Moments in time, forming a new skin.

The last thing I learn is that there is a difference between a living child and a dead one. I have no idea what Rachel might say about these stories I've shared. No way to check what she might add or want taken away. Her way of remembering the world is gone. Lost from me.

I recognize her now as wilderness. Raw. Boundless.

Where does it end? By my calculations, I left her in at least fifty places. Maybe more.

Give me a map of the world I can mark with an X for each spot.

At the summit of Black Crag, a 360-degree panorama over lakes and fells, in England's Lake District; at Yasodhara Ashram, deep in the crevasses of a gnarly log stump that looked very much like somewhere a hobbit might choose to rest; in San Francisco's Yerba Buena Gardens among a raised bed of magenta bougainvillea; at Casa Ercole, near Ancona, beneath a row of taps protruding from a baked Italian wall, the replicating shadows casting a glorious black symmetry; on the sandy cliff top at Ebey's Landing on Whidbey Island, with a view of the snow-capped Olympic Mountains for eternity; in the gaping mouths of two playground hippos along the Hudson River Parkway: Mum and baby; at Spirit Rock Meditation Centre in Marin County beneath a wooden armchair with a commemorative plaque for a man who also died young, at twenty-six years old; in a shady spot of the inner courtyard at City Palace, Udaipur, Rajasthan, and in the Rock Garden at Chandigarh, but I don't recall where, because it was crowded and I had to be quick; on the village green in Evandale, Tasmania, below the war memorial, In Memory of the Men of ANZAC; beneath a fountain-like shrub in Melbourne's Royal Botanical Gardens, its central stalk protruding skyward a generous metre, like a giant circumcised penis. I figured she'd find it suitably funny. On the freshly mowed grass overlooking Perth's Scarborough Beach, because down in the surf is where Jacquie had thrown some of Bronwen's ashes; along Tuart Walk, near Dalyellup, overtop fallen gum nuts and eucalypt leaves; along the Nimitz Way Trail in Tilden Regional Park, Berkeley; among a bed of purple crocuses blooming outside the French Canadian bakery in Nelson, BC; in Mallorca, in a sun-baked clay pot at Son Mico, a remote guesthouse overlooking the valley town of Sóller. A swag of olive branches sculpted around the pot's upper edge made me think of Rachel. She adored olives. Doubling for New Zealand, Sa Calobra, a film location in *Cloud Atlas,* was another right place. I left her at the very top — at the lookout — the road snaking ten miles down to the ocean like the ribbon path of a rhythmic gymnast; under a bench in the village of Fornalutx, the village where I made the momentous decision to fly to Australia after all.

For five months I continued to house-sit after I stopped leaving her ashes.

House-sitting worked for me. It meant being somewhere, not just seeing somewhere; geography lessons unlike those I'd learned in school. Gentle travel, I called it. There was added value, too. It was affordable. On a very limited budget, it really was the only possible way I could've lived without my own home for as long as I did.

The shifting homes, twenty-nine in all, and the views they offered (or didn't), had been a mirror to the way grief travelled inside me: sometimes coiled up tight, sometimes leaning to catch the light.

The solitary life of a house-sitter meant time for contemplation, for space to stay with my grief, often when I wished it otherwise. The social life with friends and family was noisier, and often, a great deal more fun. The balance, aloneness and togetherness, had been both invigorating and revelatory.

These homes *became* my home. And just like Rachel's ashes, they were scattered across the planet.

CHAPTER 22

Pedal Away

"Where do you live?" asks the US customs officer, wiping his brow in the blistering heat.

"North Vancouver."

It's what I always say. It's where my sister Sarah lives, where my mail's delivered, where I stay between house-sits. The closest thing to "home" as we think of it.

"Where're you heading today?"

"Seattle. I'm house-sitting for friends for a couple of weeks."

He opens the trunk, pokes around in the basket of spices, the winter coats, the suitcase. He heads off inside. Re-emerges.

"Could you pull over here please? My supervisor wants to talk with you," he says, walking off with both my Canadian and British passports. "This is going to take a while. Take a seat."

I did. For an hour.

"Problem is, you're inadmissible," he says when he returns. "You've no proof of residency in Canada or, in fact, anywhere in the world."

I remain in my chair, unsure of the correct course of action.

"Do you have something that verifies your house-sitting profile? A website?"

"I do."

He opens a notepad to a fresh page and slides it toward me. I print my blog address onto the thin blue lines.

"This could take a while longer."

"No worries," I say.

He saunters off to his cubicle. I think about my pastrami sandwich, hot and sweaty in Saran Wrap, lying there on the passenger seat, and I wish now that I'd brought it inside with me.

Take us much time as you need. He'll return to his computer, discover the About Me page on my website, and understand that my homelessness mirrored the state of my heart — the heart of a grieving mother.

Sitting in the tiny office, cool in my Australian linens, I reconciled myself to the very real possibility that I'd be denied entry. It seemed that way. So my response came as something of a revelation: whatever his decision, I could accept it. But then everything had changed my world.

I now understood that grief is not an affliction but rather something to be reconciled over time, as much in relationship with others, as with myself. I knew that grief doesn't heal us, it just changes us.

An hour later, he reappears. "I get what you're doing," he says. "You've had some stuff happen in your life." He makes a record on my file and permits me entry.

No one knows what to do with a person like me. We live collectively in homes, and someone like me who doesn't fit the mold threatens the safety of those who do. And others like me, who've chosen this life, feel chastised. Irresponsible.

But I got it. What *do* you do with someone who doesn't have a home? Even I'd begun to wonder. Why hadn't I stopped when her ashes ran out? That was March. Here I was in September.

The world shrinks back on itself when it doesn't let you pass.

How much longer would I keep living like this?

It's hard to know when to stop.

Just as it had been at the start, I couldn't name the day when I suddenly realized that I would stop. But things began to happen.

It's a glorious September day, a date the world will always remember. Twelve years ago.

The sun is up and I feel weightless.

First there is a phone call to my mother. I want her to be the first to know my news. It's news she's been waiting to hear.

For so long she's been anxious. Since I'd gone travelling, our conversations went something like this:

Mum: How are you doing? Are you okay?

Me: I'm fine. Thanks.

Mum (whining): Really?

Me (impatient): Yes! Don't I sound fine?

Mum: Well, how much longer do you plan on living like this? Don't you have to get a job?

Me: Mum, I'll stop when I'm ready.

But as time ticked on and I showed no signs of stopping, her concerns began to escalate. She was afraid that I'd vacated life entirely. What should she tell the ladies at her golf club? In her bridge group?

Grief, she believed, had a shelf life. And I, the youngest of her three daughters, was allowing it to fester. Paralyzing my future opportunities to rejoin society.

Yesterday, last night, this morning, I had made the momentous decision that after twenty-six months of living out of a suitcase, I would stop. Find a home of my own.

That morning, in the liminal space between sleep and seeing, I replayed my journey from start to finish. A journey I saw now as the adventure of a lifetime.

My mind had stopped in Tasmania. I let it stay there, indulged my memory right to the edges.

"Have you decided where you'll settle down?" she says.

"Yes. Vancouver."

"Oh, I'm so glad. Your sister will be so happy to have you back."

I felt sorely disappointed, not by my mother's joy, of course, but by the sinking sensation in my belly. The decision to move to Vancouver was a sorry compromise. I'd wrestled with it for days. It had to be Canada. Charlotte lives here. And although Vancouver held so many fearful memories, there were many happy ones too. But still, I wrestled with it. Rachel and I are entwined in the streets and buildings of Vancouver.

To rationalize my decision was to view it not as a going back, but a going forward.

"No, no, no, Mum." I nod, staccato notes. "I'm not going back."

"What do you mean?"

"Well, there's a difference. I'm not going back. I'm going to return. *Re-turn.*"

"Oh, it's all the same thing, darling. I really don't understand the difference."

It's noon by the time I strap on my helmet and pedal away. Lost in thought.

Soon I'll have a place of my own, a place to unpack those boxes I'd sealed up twenty-six months ago, give them legs.

The trail ends. Another begins. Bent on gaining speed, my wheels turn fast and easy.

The signpost: Leaving Seattle. What the heck! Enjoy it while you can.

I conjure a picture of the notes left by the homeowners, avid cyclists. "There's a great pub that we often stop at for lunch. Not sure of the name."

The floodgates open: my clothes on white hangers, my jewelry in its box, the red velvet lining cradling the few trinkets I'd chosen to keep.

I check my watch. Take my last swig of water. Three o'clock. That's when I should have turned around. Friends had invited me for dinner at 6 p.m. But in the glory of sunshine I pedal away, lost in thought.

Then it happens. My quads seize up. I stare down at my thighs, like the failing pistons of a steam engine, willing them back to life. But they're gone. I brake, try swinging a leg of fizzy jelly over the crossbar. Try walking. Try shaking the left leg, then the right.

A rider with the proper bike shorts stops.

"Is everything okay?"

"Do you need a hand?" his friend says, wheeling closer.

And I recognize their faces. These were the two men I'd spoken with earlier.

"Do you know of a pub around here?" I'd asked them. "It's where my friends stop for lunch when they bike this trail."

"No, there's not much this way," they'd said, "just a lavender farm up ahead."

And here we are again. What must I look like? A grown woman shuffling along, like a geisha.

"Oh, it's okay," I say, nodding. Pfffff. "It's nothing. I've just overdone it. Haven't ridden a bike in a long time." I smile, wave them on. "Thanks anyway."

I realize I really haven't done this in a long time; not the bike riding, but the recklessness. Nor have I thought about how my body moves. Used to move. I look down at my dead legs. Is this what it feels like when a brain tumour has its way with you? Bob had described it like a dull numbness. A pins-and-needles sluggishness.

For the next hour I interchange a stretch of walking with another of riding. I speed up in the bright sunlight (on what I find out later is the hottest September 11 on record), then pedal slowly through the shadows of sloppy trees, berating myself mercilessly. My right arm is vivid pink; I hadn't even thought to bring sunscreen.

In my mind I begin to order the events of my homecoming, never so excited to make a list. EVER. The Entering Seattle sign appears like a hallelujah chorus. With so many miles still ahead, I just want to throw the fucking bike in the bushes. I want to cry for HELP, but people don't do that. More than anything, I just want to *stop moving*.

Why didn't you stop sooner? Turn around and go home? And why so insistent on finding that pub? What's wrong with picking up a sandwich at Subway? That's what sensible people would do. But then you don't live like most sensible people. No, the rules are different for you. And you know it. Hermetically sealed in my own bubble, I play by my own rules. No need to explain, or justify my actions. No breaching any moral code. No need to pace myself.

Remember being locked inside Blake Garden? Forgetting it closed at 4 p.m.? Ignoring the telltale signs — people drifting toward the small exit gate — just so I could leave Rachel in private beneath the bench where I'd sat overlooking the Golden Gate Bridge, blinded by the yellow sky?

(I have absolutely no memory of how I got out.)

Another time in Mallorca, jolted awake. *Do you need a visa to enter Australia?* My flight was booked. I'd be leaving in two days.

And Melbourne. Dangerously late for my flight to Tasmania. Anita urged me to re-read my check-in time. I didn't. She did.

"No worries," said Anita. "We should make it there just in time."

Miss the flight and I'd have left the homeowners standing at Launceston Airport, wondering who exactly they'd agreed to hand over the keys of their property to for two months.

Why choose tension over peace? A test of self-reliance? Arrogance? Or is it nothing more than my curiosity to tempt fate? To discover, perhaps, how I might handle a critical event that wasn't about someone dying?

Yes. That's it, isn't it? That's when I felt it, that aliveness: forcing a drama, some pivotal event to shake me up, free of the mundane, the predictable. No, I'd had a taste of dying and I was hooked.

Imagine lying beside your lover, or holding the hand of your daughter. Both are close to death. Love is the current, and together you are drowning.

Hold tight. It's almost time. Only one of you — we both know which one — will come up for air.

No one dare use the word seductive to describe the end of life. But there it is.

To be so hollowed out and so full at the same time. Craving it to be over and yet to go on forever. What a terrible discovery.

Is this what I'm doing here? Attempting to replicate what used to be us? What's now just me? Is this why I can't stop? Why I crave these "on the edge" moments? Moments that allow these altered states to happen?

Perhaps. But then might it also be a celebration of life? Of living? Of imagining the joy they'd feel in my aliveness?

Because this grief thing I know, above and beyond all else, can produce an equally powerful force — gratitude. Gratitude for what I have, not for what I don't, and it comes from knowing how exquisitely fragile life is. It came to me first, like a violent wave, after Bob died. Flooded through me on this journey.

This is not a gift. Simply a by-product that supports the cause-and-effect Newtonian logic: for every action there is an equal and opposite reaction.

Scoff all you want, but I'm right about this.

CHAPTER 23

ONE BOX

Stopping demands a different courage. Becoming visible again, and accountable, makes me afraid. Can I re-emerge a full citizen of the world? Or have I been away too long?

Home. Just imagining it makes my heart skip. One morning I catch my hand trembling as I squeeze paste along the bristles of my toothbrush. Another time a rising nausea makes me stop the car.

What will bear the mark of my time? *That versus this?* Won't an address simply serve to reduce my life to a street number and name, as if the entire journey no longer mattered?

How will I keep unfamiliarity my companion while living in familiar surroundings?

Will settling down mean settling for?

And will I, God forbid, get attached to my stuff? To everything in its right place? It happens.

Without question my life will shift: *extraordinary to ordinary.*

Will I continue to see the gift in days? Extend the same kindness to those who are lost? Thank cooks and counter staff in cafés and shops? Call them by name, just as Bob had? My intuitive grasp for telling people how much I appreciate their time, their friendship, their kindness, can I sustain it?

I've come to like this woman. This woman of wings. I've grown loyal to her ways. I'd hate to abandon her.

But the worst thing about stopping is this: Nothing lies ahead. There is nowhere to go next. Nothing to do.

It's fall. Things are dying. I rent a fifth-floor corner apartment in Kitsilano. Even on the darkest days I see mostly sky. It's vast in every direction. Open and watery.

Burrard Inlet separates me from a landscape of loss: North Vancouver, the place I called home for almost thirty years. The Lions Gate Bridge is more a buffer than a link. Still, the transition feels perilous. I commit to a year.

I take back the box from Daryl. A red Ikea box in which I'd packed up her life.

One box.

It's a foggy day. Late October. My back against the comfy chair, I take a seat on the freshly varnished hardwood floor. I'm wearing the grey sweats I'd bought for her twenty-third — and final — birthday.

I remove the lid.

On the top is a printed copy of an email sent to Daryl from Michael Henderson, the glider pilot from Nevada.

You may remember while you were here last November the glider that was at the last stage of restoration. The glider Rachel compared herself to. Well, we got her out to fly yesterday. This week we'll paint the wingtips. Black and maroon racing stripes will be added to the fuselage. But today we let it sit there so we could look at her one more time. The History Channel film team will be here next week to make that glider the star of the show for a March airing. With your permission, we would like to add a cursive "RACHEL" to the outside front seat entry. That's what we will call it, instead of "898," for the rest of its existence. From now on Rachel's name will be mentioned every time she gets flown. Promise.

Unforgettable Places to See Before You Die is where I left it, close to the top.

I hold the book with both hands. The cover, I'd never liked. Nor had Rachel. The promise of far-off lands, we agreed, deserved better. I flip through the book like a Vegas card shuffler. The Taj Mahal is close to the beginning. I pull out a pen from my handbag, the one I bought in Carmel, rotate the tip.

I draw a star, the kind Rachel drew, practising first on the back of my hand. Rachel's stars had five points. Mine: six. The star would have to be perfect, as if she'd come home and drawn it herself.

I flip through her travel journal. Find this.

July 1/2007
Happy Canada Day! Ferry got into Bari around 9ish, went to the train station with everyone, the girls went to Naples, the guys to Rome, and me to Bologna, then transfer to Florence. I basically spent the whole day on the train. East coast of Italy is very beautiful — great beaches and bright turquoise blue water.

I check my own journal, pull it from a box marked "Journals."

July 1, 2010, was the date I first released her ashes, on a beach in Italy. Exactly three years earlier, she'd passed that beach on the train.

I clamber to my feet, move to the window, and look out over English Bay. Freighters dot the water. Gulls circle and squawk. Two crows — always two — poised on a wire. I watch as one preens the other, burying its beak deep beneath the glossy black.

Here I am.

I lift the latch and slide the window open. Lean out slightly. A cool gust of wind blasts my face.

Where, I wonder, is she?

My daughter, swallowed up in Earth's mighty belly. Travelling on a mystery tour that I created.

She once belonged in every home I made for her. Those homes, now, are too many to name or know. Tucked into empty spaces, adrift at sea, sunk in wet dirt, feeding plants and trees that will still be growing after I'm gone.

For twenty-six months we travelled together. Carrying each other. She helped me find beauty in out-of-the-way places, taught me grace in living with uncertainty.

There's so much to learn from travel, and endings, and children. Changing geography. Solitude. Silence. Timeless days. They accrue.

Some things cannot be fixed. They can only be carried and shared.

Her ashes scattered in the world became my world. How much more union can there be?

She's learned, by now, to go her own way. I am learning to find mine.

The crows fly away; first one, then eventually, the other. Out on the street I see my neighbour walking down to the beach, her thick white hair pulled up in a bun. I close the window, put on my shoes and head out to join her.

Acknowledgements

Thank you to the homeowners around the world who trusted me with their front door key, and the generous friends who welcomed me to stay. There were many.

The entire community at Hollyburn Elementary School who rallied around me: thank you.

Betsy Warland at Vancouver Manuscript Intensive, my extraordinary mentor. The book is far better for her astute comments than anything I could have accomplished alone. Thanks to the Claire Festel Scholarship and Carl Leggo for inspiration.

This book would not have existed without Caitlin Press. Vici Johnstone, Holly Vestad, Christine Savage and Michael Despotovic, thank you for your steadfast support. My editor, Yvonne Blomer, for finding the structure I couldn't. My agent, Morty Mint, for his calm confidence.

Irene Mock envisioned this book before I did and supported me all the way. Thank you to early readers Verna Relkoff and Tara McGuire. Shannon Leone Fowler and Zoe Grams for your bounty of help.

My parents and sisters, who watched over me while I rebuilt my life. My family of friends who have looked after me in a million ways: Jenny, Saskia, James, Richard, Julie, Petra, Pauline, Adrian and Meg. I could not begin to list all you have done.

Charlotte, for you I reserve my most profound love and gratitude. My darling Bob. And, of course, Rachel, this book is for you.